OXFORD MEDICAL PUBLICATIONS

Handbook of Child Nutrition
(SECOND EDITION)

?6

Keep 18
June 18
LA

Handbook of Child Nutrition

....

SECOND EDITION

B.L. WARDLEY

*Department of Pediatrics, University of Medicine and Dentistry,
Robert Wood Johnson Medical School, New Jersey, USA*

J.W.L. PUNTIS

*Department of Paediatrics and Child Health, The University of Leeds
and The General Infirmary at Leeds, UK*

and

L.S. TAITZ

Oxford   New York   Tokyo

OXFORD UNIVERSITY PRESS

1997

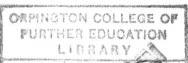
Oxford University Press, Great Clarendon Street, Oxford OX2 6DP
Oxford New York
Athens Auckland Bangkok Bogota Bombay Buenos Aires
Calcutta Cape Town Dar es Salaam Delhi Florence Hong Kong
Istanbul Karachi Kuala Lumpur Madras Madrid Melbourne
Mexico City Nairobi Paris Singapore Taipei Tokyo Toronto Warsaw
and associated companies in
Berlin Ibadan

Oxford is a trade mark of Oxford University Press

Published in the United States
by Oxford University Press Inc., New York

© Wardley, Puntis, and Taitz, 1997

A catalogue record for this book is available from the British Library

Library of Congress Cataloging in Publication Data
Wardley, B. L. (Bridget L.)
Handbook of child nutrition / Bridget Wardley, J. W. L. Puntis,
Leonard Taitz. – 2nd ed.
Main entry of previous ed. under Taitz.
Includes bibliographical references and index.
1. Children–Nutrition. 2. Children–Diseases–Nutritional
aspects. I. Puntis, J. W. L. (John W. L.) II. Taitz, Leonard S.
III. Title
RJ206.W28   1997   613.2´083–dc21   97-12677
ISBN 0 19 262787 2 (Hbk)
ISBN 0 19 262786 4 (Pbk)

Typeset by Newgen Imaging Systems, India

Printed in Great Britain by Biddles Ltd, Guildford and Kings Lynn

Foreword

Not so many years ago a professed interest in Child Nutrition would have seemed quaint. Now it is a burgeoning topic seen to be related not only to growth but also to behaviour, immunity, adult life, and so on.

The first edition of this book was published during the 'quaint phase' but even then it made its mark among health professionals concerned with children.

This new edition has emulated the first and brought innovation. It encompasses the 'nutritional nuts and bolts' of child health as seen in hospital, in the community, and in the child's home. Moreover it sets them in a firm amalgam of experience and scientific rationale—a rare and, in the hands of these authors, an effective combination.

Dr Brian Wharton
Director-General
British Nutrition Foundation

Preface

First published in 1989, this book has been updated to take into account some of the many changes in the field of paediatric nutrition which have taken place since that time. Written by a paediatric dietitian and paediatric gastroenterologist who together have pooled their knowledge and experience, the text provides a balance of dietetic and medical opinion forming a practical and compact handbook of child nutrition.

Parents have many questions about diet and nutrition and require accurate and sensible advice from health professionals. This book aims to be a suitable guide for health visitors, community nurses, midwives, general practitioners, and others who have no special knowledge of nutrition and dietetics but who have to deal with dietary problems in the course of their work. It also serves as a useful introduction to paediatric nutrition for dietetic, medical, and nursing students whilst remaining accessible to the interested lay person.

The second edition now includes sections on growth in children, feeding the premature infant, enteral tube feeding, and parenteral nutrition with particular reference to feeding methods in the community. We have also expanded the discussion of chronic diseases which require special nutritional intervention. 'Bullet' lists have been provided to focus the reader on concise practical information relating to different topics and at the end of each chapter we have included a short list of references for those requiring more detailed knowledge. A list of self-help groups and further sources of information appear at the end of the book. Sadly, Leonard Taitz died after the publication of the first edition of this book. We gratefully acknowledge the fact that so much of his expertise and enthusiasm can be found in the second edition.

We would like to thank many colleagues who have provided us with useful feedback on the content, including the dietitians at

Sheffield Children's Hospital, Dr Brian Wharton, Mrs Anita MacDonald, and Dr Mary Rudolph. We also wish to thank our families for their support and for teaching us that feeding is much more than nutrition!

New Jersey   B.L.W.
Leeds   J.W.L.P.
June 1997

Contents

1 **Assessment of growth in children**   1

The use of growth charts   1
Anthropometry and evaluation of growth   9

2 **Infant feeding**   15

Feeding sucklings—breast feeding   15
Feeding sucklings—formula feeding   37
Feeding weanlings   45
Feeding the preterm infant   48

3 **The preschoolchild**   54

A balanced diet for the toddler   56
The child who 'won't eat'   58
Bizarre diets   61
Iron deficiency anaemia   61
Are supplementary vitamins necessary?   62
Nutrients 'at risk'   63
Toddler diarrhoea   64
Constipation   67
Dental caries   70

4 **The schoolchild and adolescent**   73

A balanced diet for the schoolchild   73
Nutritional issues in schoolchildren   76
School meals   79
Diet and behaviour   81
The adolescent   83
Nutritional issues in adolescence   84

5 **Healthy eating to prevent adult disease**   88

The health of the nation   89
Cardio-vascular disease   91

Salt and hypertension   98
Diet and the general population   99
Principles for good eating   102
The 'Barker hypothesis'   104
Iron deficiency   106
Bone disease   108
Cancer   110

6   Cultural and ethnic diets   113
Vegetarian diets   114
Cult diets   121
Diets of different ethnic origins   125

7   Feeding problems in infants   130
Failure to thrive in breast-fed babies   130
Delay in establishment of breast milk supply   131
Jaundice   132
Fears about 'hypoglycaemia'   132
Breast-feeding problems   133
Possiting   135
Vomiting   138
Colic   140
Wind   141
Constipation   142
Choking episodes   144
Overfeeding and underfeeding   145
Errors in bottle-feeding technique   146
Babies who are difficult to feed   146
Force-feeding   149
The dissatisfied baby   150

8   Diarrhoea   157
Acute diarrhoea   157
Chronic diarrhoea   164
'Diarrhoea de retour'   164

9   Food allergy   166
Food intolerance   167
Cow's milk protein intolerance   170

Diagnosing food allergies 172
Dietary treatment of food intolerance 175
Eczema 178
Coeliac disease 180
Non-allergic food intolerance 182
Food 'allergy' in less well defined situations 186

10 Obesity 191

Prevalence of obesity 192
Causes of obesity 193
Consequences of childhood obesity 197
Dietary treatment 199
Behaviour modification 204
Preventing childhood obesity 205

11 Dietary management of metabolic disorders 208

Inborn errors of metabolism 210
Hyperlipidaemia 212
Cystic fibrosis 214
Phenylketonuria 216
Organic acidaemias 219
Galactosaemia 220
Glycogen storage disease 222
Diabetes mellitus 223
Ketogenic diet for epilepsy 226

12 Nutritional management in chronic disease 228

Enteral tube feeding 229
Parenteral feeding 229
Home nutritional support 230
Gastrostomy feeding 233
Home parenteral nutrition 237
Specific disorders commonly requiring
  nutritional intervention 238
Liver disease 238
Inflammatory bowel disease 240
Renal disease 242
Human immunodeficiency virus infection 245
Cancer 247

Further reading and references   249

Self-help groups   250

Organizations offering nutrition information   251

Index   253

1

....

Assessment of growth in children

An understanding of normal growth is essential for all health professionals working with children and accurate anthropometric assessment is important for monitoring growth and nutritional status. A complete nutritional assessment includes a dietary history, anthropometric measurements, and biochemical evaluation and in this chapter we give a brief overview of growth and anthropometric assessment in children. Various other aspects of nutritional assessment are discussed in different sections of the book. However, a more detailed discussion of this subject is beyond the scope of this book and the reader is referred to the excellent reviews found in the reference section at the end of this chapter and also to the further reading section at the end of the book.

The use of growth charts

The growth and maturation of the infant and child progress at different rates. In the first year of life a baby will triple his birth weight and increase in length by 50%. After one year of age growth slows down, but continues at a more steady rate until the start of puberty, when increases in growth hormone initiate a final and rapid growth spurt.

Accurate measurement and the use of standard growth charts are important tools for monitoring a child's progress. Clinics and GPs surgeries must have well maintained equipment appropriate for children and staff should receive training in order to ensure consistent, accurate measurements. Growth charts are compiled from measurements of large numbers of babies and children. The data are usually cross-sectional, being obtained from different sets of infants, rather than longitudinal when measurements at each age are from the same set of children observed over time. The value of centile charts is that infants and children can usually be expected to follow a genetically predetermined centile line without much deviation upwards or downwards. However there are some important qualifications to this assumption.

Well-constructed, standard, current centile charts should be used. New growth charts (Fig. 1.1) are now available in Britain, and are known as the '1990 nine centile United Kingdom charts'. They are based on growth surveys between 1978 and 1990, reflecting more current infant feeding practices and the different growth patterns of breast-fed infants. These charts differ from the older Tanner and Whitehouse charts in several ways and nine centiles are now given, the lowest being the 0.4 line. Only one child in 250 will fall below this line, therefore making this lowest centile a clear cut indicator for referral. The new charts also allow for plotting the growth of the preterm infant. When using the growth charts, referral for further investigation is recommended under the following circumstances:

• height below the 0.4 centile
• weight below the 0.4 centile
• height above the 99.6 centile
• weight above the 99.6 centile
• a crossing of two centiles between two annual measurements.

Centiles for height are remarkably consistent and any change in the position of height centile is a matter for remark. This consistency which has come to be called 'tracking' is probably a reflection of the strong genetic influence on height.

Although weight centiles also tend to track consistently, short-term deviations are more common than for height. This is because

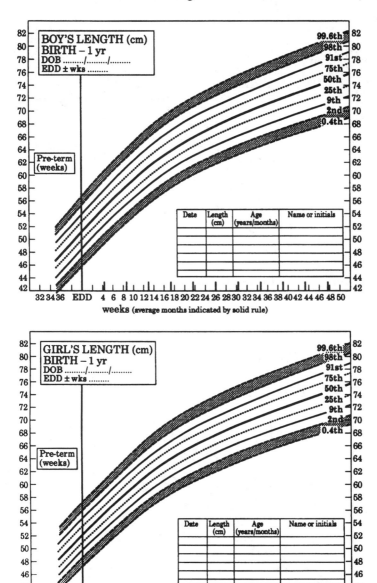

Fig. 1.1. Growth charts for boys and girls. © Child Growth Foundation, London.

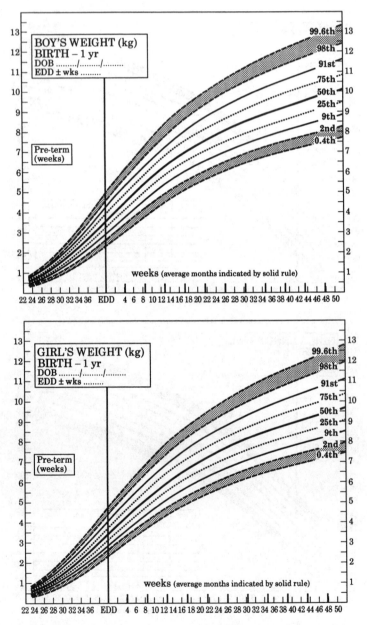

Fig. 1.1. (*Continued*). © Child Growth Foundation, London.

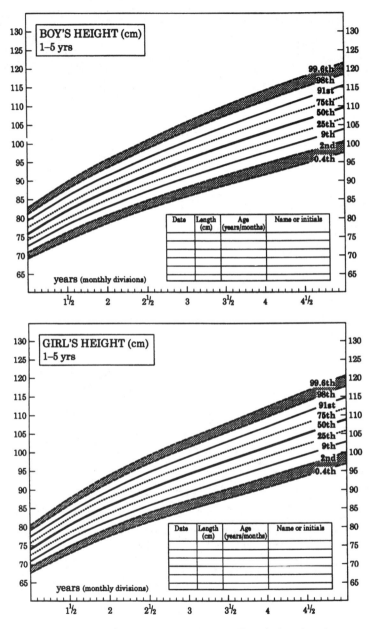

Fig. 1.1. (*Continued*). © Child Growth Foundation, London.

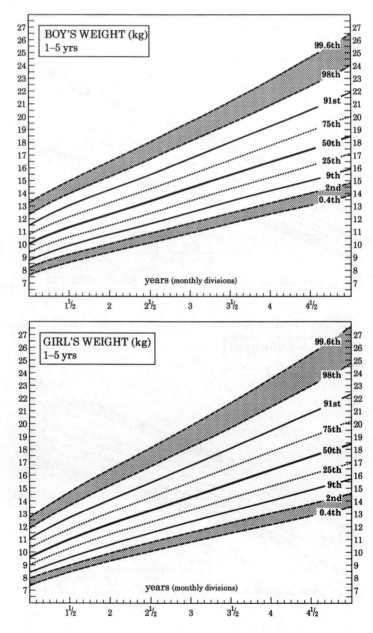

Fig. 1.1. (*Continued*). © Child Growth Foundation, London.

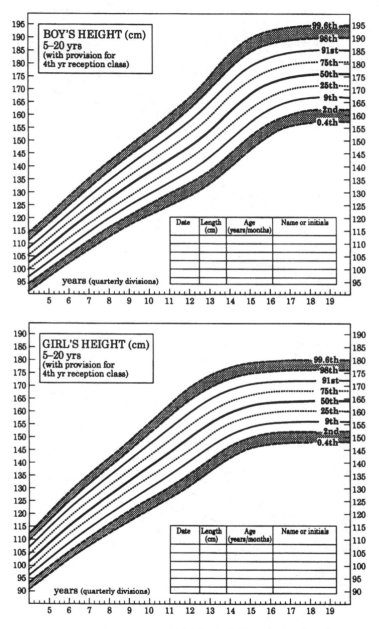

Fig. 1.1. (*Continued*). © Child Growth Foundation, London.

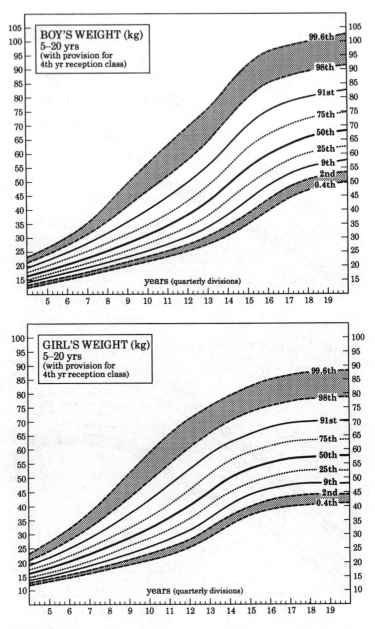

Fig. 1.1. (*Continued*). © Child Growth Foundation, London.

environmental influences have a more powerful effect and possibly because the range of weight gain patterns is intrinsically more variable. This is particularly true for the first six months of life.

Special growth charts are available for some groups of children including Down syndrome and should be used when appropriate.

Normal babies who do not follow centile charts

The newborn infant has spent nine months in utero, which is an extremely influential environment. Thus weight at birth is the measurement least likely to reflect genetic predisposition. It is therefore not surprising that some babies show an early deviation from birth weight centile and follow a new centile.

Some infants are relatively small for their gestational age. If a baby who was genetically intended to be on the 91st centile has some degree of intra-uterine malnutrition then birth weight may be on the 50th centile. A period of very rapid weight gain sometimes follows as the baby undergoes 'catch up' growth (Fig. 1.2). On the other hand, an infant born on the 91st centile because some maternal factor has caused it to lay down excess adipose tissue, may in shedding it, lower his centile position.

The interpretation of centile charts in the early months of life can be difficult and the majority of babies who change centiles turn out to be normal. When in doubt it is wise to seek the help of a paediatrician who will often simply follow and repeat measurements if the baby is otherwise well. If centiles continue to be crossed, further investigation may be indicated, but in the absence of other clinical features these are almost invariably negative. One should always bear in mind the possibility that growth failure may be a manifestation of complex psycho-social factors in the family.

Anthropometry and evaluation of growth

When concern regarding growth prompts referral to a paediatrician, a detailed evaluation of nutritional status should be performed. This will include an assessment of growth as well as other nutritional parameters such as dietary intake, feeding history, and biochemical assessment. The three basic measures used for assessing growth status in children are age, weight, and

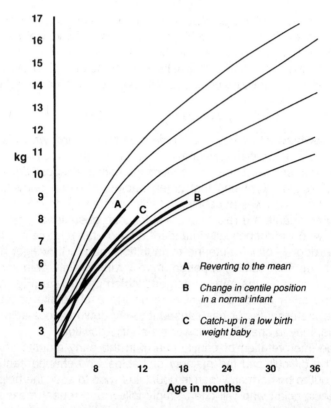

Fig. 1.2. Examples of normal weight changes in infants.

height. These are combined, compared with reference standards (growth charts) and expressed as the following indices:

• height-for-age
• weight-for-age
• weight-for-height.

These measurements should be made by a trained and practiced professional according to standard protocols. In interpreting growth status some useful classifications are:

• low height-for-age (stunting; < 3rd centile) which is an indication of chronic malnutrition

- low weight-for-height (wasting; < 80% expected weight-for-height) usually the result of acute malnutrition.

It is also important to consider other causes of growth failure as well as malnutrition when assessing the child. Weight may be influenced by dehydration, fluid retention, ascites, and tumour mass, making weight-for-height a potentially inaccurate index of nutritional status.

When there are other factors affecting body weight different methods of anthropometric assessment can be used. Arm anthropometry is a useful and simple tool in children, and mid-upper arm circumference (MUAC) has been shown to correlate well with weight-for-height and can substitute for this in assessing acute malnutrition.

Anthropometric ratios

To interpret anthropometric data various measurements are combined in different ratios and compared to standards. These ratios include weight/height^2 (body mass index [BMI]); weight/height^3; MUAC/height; MUAC/upper arm length; MUAC/head circumference. All these ratios relate one measurement which is likely to be affected by acute malnutrition to another which is not; however, in chronic malnutrition both measures can be affected and a misleadingly 'normal' ratio results.

At the opposite end of the nutritional spectrum there are unresolved difficulties with defining obesity in childhood. There is no generally accepted definition which differentiates between normal or healthy fatness and that which has negative implications for health. The body mass index (BMI) is widely used in adults, and > 30 kg/m^2 is associated with significant risk of increased mortality. In childhood, however, the amount of fat tissue varies at different ages which means that BMI also varies and centile charts which refer to age related norms are necessary to interpret this ratio. An agreed definition of obesity in children has not as yet been developed (see Chapter 10), but any child with a BMI above the 99.6th centile should be referred to a paediatrician. Standard BMI charts for children are available (Fig. 1.3),

Referral guidelines

Consider referral for any boy whose BMI falls above the 99.6th centile/below the 0.4th centile as significantly over/underweight even on the basis of a single measurement. It is possible that a boy whose BMI falls in the tinted areas should also be referred. However, during infancy large but transient changes in centile may occur due to the shape of the charts, and these changes are normal. It should be remembered that the earlier the age of the second rise, the greater the risk of future obesity. Remember also that while BMI has a high correlation with relative fatness or leanness it is actually assessing the weight-to-height relationship: **this may give misleading results in boys who are very stocky and muscular who might appear obese on the BMI alone.**

BOYS

BMI CHART
(BIRTH - 20 YEARS)
United Kingdom cross-sectional reference data : 1995/1

Name...

NHS No. ☐☐☐ ☐☐☐ ☐☐☐☐

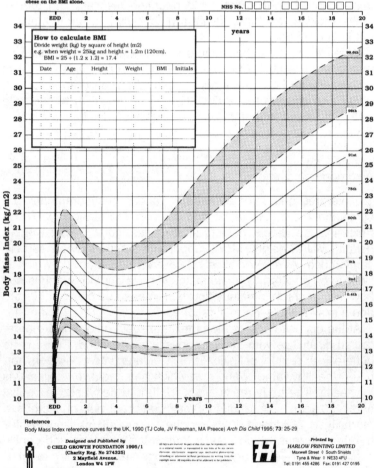

How to calculate BMI

Divide weight (kg) by square of height (m2)
e.g. when weight = 25kg and height = 1.2m (120cm),
BMI = 25 ÷ (1.2 x 1.2) = 17.4

Date	Age	Height	Weight	BMI	Initials
: :	: :	: :	:	:	:
: :	: :	: :	:	:	:
: :	: :	: :	:	:	:
: :	: :	: :	:	:	:
: :	: :	: :	:	:	:
: :	: :	: :	:	:	:

Reference
Body Mass Index reference curves for the UK, 1990 (TJ Cole, JV Freeman, MA Preece) *Arch Dis Child* 1995; **73**: 25-29

Designed and Published by
© **CHILD GROWTH FOUNDATION** 1995/1
(Charity Reg. No 274325)
2 Mayfield Avenue,
London W4 1PW

Printed by
HARLOW PRINTING LIMITED
Maxwell Street ◊ South Shields
Tyne & Wear ◊ NE33 4PU
Tel: 0191 455 4286 Fax: 0191 427 0195

Fig. 1.3. Body mass index charts. © Child Growth Foundation, London.

Referral guidelines

Consider referral for any girl whose BMI falls above the 99.6th centile/below the 0.4th centile as significantly over/underweight even on the basis of a single measurement. It is possible that a girl whose BMI falls in the tinted areas should also be referred. However, during infancy large but transient changes in centile may occur due to the shape of the charts, and these changes are normal. It should be remembered that the earlier the age of the second rise, the greater the risk of future obesity. Remember also that while BMI has a high correlation with relative fatness or leanness it is actually assessing the weight-to-height relationship: **this may give misleading results in girls who are very stocky and muscular who might appear obese on the BMI alone.**

GIRLS
BMI CHART
(BIRTH - 20 YEARS)
United Kingdom cross-sectional reference data : 1995/1

Name..

NHS No.

How to calculate BMI

Divide weight (kg) by square of height (m2)
e.g. when weight = 25kg and height = 1.2m (120cm).
BMI = 25 ÷ (1.2 x 1.2) = 17.4

Date	Age	Height	Weight	BMI	Initials
: :	: :	: :	: :	: :	: :
: :	: :	: :	: :	: :	: :
: :	: :	: :	: :	: :	: :
: :	: :	: :	: :	: :	: :
: :	: :	: :	: :	: :	: :
: :	: :	: :	: :	: :	: :

Body Mass Index (kg/m2)

Reference

Body Mass Index reference curves for the UK, 1990 (TJ Cole, JV Freeman, MA Preece) *Arch Dis Child* 1995; **73**: 25-29

Designed and Published by
© CHILD GROWTH FOUNDATION 1995/1
(Charity Reg. No 274325)
2 Mayfield Avenue,
London W4 1PW

Printed by
HARLOW PRINTING LIMITED
Maxwell Street ◊ South Shields
Tyne & Wear ◊ NE33 4PU
Tel: 0191 455 4286 Fax: 0191 427 0195

Fig. 1.3. (*Continued*). © Child Growth Foundation, London.

and provide an additional assessment tool when used in conjunction with growth charts.

Understanding data from groups of children

Sometimes it is necessary to examine nutritional status in groups of children of both sexes and different ages, an example being when assessing the impact of a particular dietary intervention on nutritional status, such as a period of elemental diet in Crohn's disease. This can be done by comparing measurements from an individual with the standards for a child of the same sex and age. A number that is meaningful for each member of the group without further reference to age or sex can be derived. The usual way of doing this is to classify by centile range, express as a percentage of the median and then as a standard deviation score, known as a z-score. Changes in z-score before and after the intervention can then be compared. The reference standards most widely used for z-scores are those from the United States Centre for Health Statistics (NCHS). In practice there are some difficulties with these scores and care must be taken to make appropriate interpretations.

Further reading

Hall, D.M.B. (1995). Monitoring children's growth: new charts will help. *British Medical Journal*, **311**, 583–4.

Poskitt, E.M.E (1995). Defining childhood obesity: the relative body mass index (BMI). *Acta Paediatrica*, **84**, 961–3.

Scott, B.J., Artman, H., and Sachiko, S.T. (1992). Growth assessment in children: A review. *Topics in Clinical Nutrition*, **8**(1), 5–31.

Smith, D.E. and Booth, I.W. (1989). Nutritional assessment of children: guidelines on collecting and interpreting anthropometric data. *Journal of Human Nutrition and Dietetics*, **2**, 217–24.

Tanner, J.M. and Kelnar, C.J.H. (1992). Physical growth, development and puberty. In *Textbook of Paediatrics* (ed. Forfar and Arneil) (4th edn). pp. 389–424. Churchill Livingstone, Edinburgh.

World Health Organisation (1983). *Measuring change in nutritional status*. Guidelines for assessing the nutritional impact of supplementary feeding programmes for vulnerable groups. *World Health Organisation*, Geneva.

2

....

Infant feeding

The principles for the successful feeding of the overwhelming majority of infants and children are now well understood and although isolated problems remain there is no reason why almost all babies and children should not be correctly fed and nourished. It is conventional to make a distinction between those infants who still depend largely on milk as their source of nutrition (sucklings) and those who eat mainly solid foods (toddlers). During the transitional intervening phase, it is convenient to describe the babies as weanlings.

Feeding sucklings

Breast-feeding

Breast-feeding on demand remains the ideal form of feeding for healthy babies who are born at term. The reasons for continuing to accept this philosophy are well set out in official statements and the World Health Organisation accepts that the vast majority of women (97% or more) are capable of breast-feeding. In the UK, of the 63% of women who breast-feed their newborn infants only a few (26%) are still fully breast-feeding at four months. The needs of the young infant are constantly changing (Table 2.1). Human milk is a remarkably variable food and not only evolves during the period of lactation to meet the needs of the baby during the early months of life, but also changes according to mothers diet. These first 4–6 months are a period of very rapid growth and development particularly for the brain. The amino acid and fatty acid composition of breast milk is ideally suited to meet these needs.

Suckling a baby at the breast can also have important emotional effects on the mother–child relationship. It seems likely that attachment of the mother to her baby is assisted both by the close physical contact and by the pleasure which successful breast-feeding evokes. Some of the many other benefits are listed below.

For baby:
- ideal nutritional composition
- protective factors:
    active enzymes to help digestion
    immunoglobulins to prevent infection
    hormones and growth factors
- fewer respiratory and gastrointestinal infections
- reduced risk of ear infections
- helps jaw and tooth development
- reduced risk of some chronic diseases
- protects against allergy
- improved neurological, visual, and oral development

For mother:
- inexpensive and convenient
- promotes good bonding between mother and infant
- uterus contracts faster
- conservation of iron stores; less anaemia
- possible health benefits include reduced risk of breast cancer and osteoporosis
- mother often feels better and has a higher self-esteem.

Although breast milk is ideal for most infants, there are a few absolute contra-indications including galactosaemia, alactasia (congenital absence of the gut enzyme lactase), and certain

Table 2.1. Reference nutrient intakes of selected nutrients for infants

Nutrient	0–3 months		4–6 months		7–9 months		10–12 months	
	male	female	male	female	male	female	male	female
Energy (EAR)								
kcal	545	515	690	645	825	765	920	865
Protein (g)	12.5		12.7		13.7		14.9	
Thiamin (mg)	0.2		0.2		0.2		0.3	
Riboflavin (mg)	0.4		0.4		0.4		0.4	
Folate (µg)	50		50		50		50	
Vitamin C (mg)	25		25		25		25	
Vitamin A (µg)	350		350		350		350	
Vitamin D (µg)	8.5		8.5		7		7	
Calcium (mmol)	13.1 (525 mg)		13.1 (525 mg)		13.1 (525 mg)		13.1 (525 mg)	
Iron (µg)	30 (1.7 mg)		80 (4.3 mg)		140 (7.8 mg)		140 (7.8 mg)	

EAR: estimated average requirement

(Adapted from: Department of Health (1991). Report on health and social subjects. *Dietary reference values for food, energy and nutrients for the United Kingdom*. Report No. 41, HMSO, UK)

drugs which the mother may have to take during the lactation period which cross into breast milk. Breast-feeding is also contra-indicated for mothers using addictive drugs such as cocaine or who consume large amounts of alcohol. Currently mothers who are infected with HIV are recommended not to breast-feed because of the risk of transmitting this to the infant. In the developing world, in countries where large numbers of women are now HIV-positive, breast-feeding is still recommended because it offers protection against the high incidence of infectious disease and malnutrition, both major causes of death.

Most mothers who genuinely wish to breast-feed their babies are able to overcome minor problems with suitable support. Many of those who give up may not have been fully committed to do so in the first place and were perhaps not given sufficient support and encouragement to continue. The most important factors which determine the prevalence of breast-feeding are motivation and support by health care professionals and parental motivation. There is a need for health education at school and the development of a general climate of support for breast-feeding. Breast-feeding remains a social-class related phenomenon, heavily slanted towards the older and more educated section of the community. It is particularly disturbing that the rate of breast-feeding appears to have fallen among younger first-time mothers and those not educated beyond the age of 18. The general decline in breast-feeding rates may be related to the increasing numbers of women who return to work earlier. Mothers who do not breast-feed their firstborns are unlikely to breast-feed subsequent infants.

Breast-feeding is not an entirely instinctive process and mothers, particularly those breast-feeding for the first time require a great deal of help, support, and encouragement during the early stages. As the vast majority of babies are now born in hospital it is here that this process must begin with encouragement of demand feeding and avoidance of artificial teats and pacifiers (dummies). Supplementary feeds or drinks of dextrose water must not be given unless medically indicated and rooming in should be encouraged, allowing mothers and infants to remain together 24 hours a day.

Continued support at home is also necessary. This is initially provided by the midwife and later by the health visitor. This dual system of care is desirable for several reasons but does have the potential for the giving of conflicting advice. Midwives and health visitors need to be knowledgeable about the practicalities of breast-feeding, should communicate with each other and ensure that they share a common philosophy. Failure to work together frequently causes difficulty, particularly if the mother is also being given advice by general practitioners, community doctors, or paediatricians. This conflict may arise from genuine differences of opinion, hence the importance of establishing infant feeding policies and guidelines which are agreed upon by all concerned.

Help and constructive support may also come from friends or relatives who have breast-fed their own babies and there are a number of support groups which give help and advice to breast-feeding mothers; these include the National Childbirth Trust and the La Leche League. The family attitude to breast-feeding is very important for its success. An unsupportive father or sceptical grandparent can stop a mother from breast-feeding.

During the last ten years, after a rapid rise in breast-feeding nationally, the proportion of mothers breast-feeding at six weeks has stabilized at around 40% and more recently appears to have declined again. The recent decline in breast-feeding is cause for concern, but probably originates in attitudes which have become established long before pregnancy. Women who are determined to breast-feed usually succeed. While it is important that mothers who start breast-feeding their babies should be given all the support and advice they need, it seems that those who favour more breast-feeding (health professionals) will need to concentrate their efforts on educating the young would-be parents from less privileged social class groups into believing that it is desirable.

Establishing lactation

Attachment Newborn infants are endowed with limited innate behaviour consisting mainly of survival reflexes such as head turning, startle, and grasp. Among these are two reflexes associated with feeding—the ability to suck and swallow and the rooting reflex. These are present in all but preterm infants of less than 32 weeks gestation. Curiously, the ability to fix at the nipple does not appear to be inborn and infants vary considerably in the speed with which they learn the trick. This is to a considerable extent determined by the skill of the person who assists the mother with the first feeds.

Successful attachment appears to be influenced by several factors:

• the state of mind of the mother
• the degree of alertness of the baby
• the timing of the first feed.
• the positioning of the baby at the breast.

A difficult struggle at this time can have a devastating effect on the mother's morale and may be an important factor in later success of lactation. A gentle and supportive assistant can make all the difference. The suggestion that voluntary agencies have a role to play in this has always been resisted by many professionals. It is also questionable whether busy maternity units are ideal place for this delicate and personal event. Fortunately most babies are obliging, learn quickly, and are soon adept at the art.

The first days   At birth, milk production is close to zero because of the inhibiting effect of placental oestrogen. The removal of the placenta results in a sudden stimulus to production of colostrum but the volume is very low. The energy content is well below even the lower needs of the newborn infant. The metabolic rate of newborn infants is low but increases rapidly during the first week of life so that energy consumption almost doubles. It is thus inevitable that breast-fed babies will lose some weight during the first days of life. The colostrum is, of course, important for its antibody content and the presence of other humoral agents. The very low energy intake acts as a feeding stimulus to the baby who will be predisposed to suck vigorously when put to the breast. This in turn is a key stimulus for increasing milk production, first by leading to the release of oxytocin which causes contraction of myo-epithelial cells in the milk ducts propelling milk out of the breast and second, by stimulating production of prolactin which in turn stimulates the formation and maturation of the milk (Fig. 2.1).

In addition to these direct effects, oxytocin may be inducing pleasure in the mother, re-inforcing the desire to breast-fed, while prolactin acts as a suppressor of ovulation.

Positioning With successful establishment of lactation a supply of milk begins to flow, which increases with the needs of the baby. These favourable events presuppose that the healthy, hungry baby will be put to the breast at frequent intervals. A crucial component of this whole process is the need for the baby to suck at the breast and for this to be successful, correct positioning is vital. The baby should be facing the mother's breast so that

Reflexes involved in the establishment of breast milk secretion

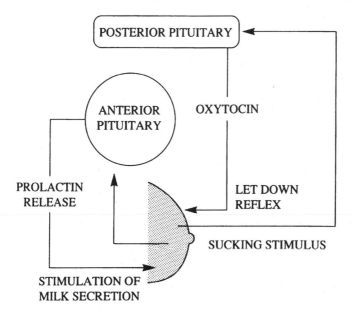

Fig. 2.1. Reflexes involved in the establishment of breast milk secretion.

the baby's neck is not twisted, a helpful description of this position is 'belly to belly' (Fig. 2.2). The baby's mouth will gape wide in response to the rooting reflex to accept the nipple and it is important that the baby takes in the nipple and much of the areola to form a 'teat'. The lower lip should be turned out and the tongue under the mothers nipple. The suck cycle is very important in the establishment of breast-feeding and is quite different to the technique required for bottle-feeding. Rapid sucking, followed by slower, rhythmic sucking and swallowing, will stimulate the let-down reflex and a rapid flow of milk commences.

There are a number of positions in which the baby can be fed, good attachment is important in all and the mother may require assistance initially. Whatever the position chosen the mother should be comfortable and supported with pillows if necessary, with the baby's back and head also given support.

Frequency and length of breast-feeds   The interval between feeds will vary with different infants and will also change over time. It may also be different at various times of day, for example a baby may feed every two hours in the evening but four hourly at other times during the day. Some babies will require feeding every two hours, especially in the early days, whereas others will feed every three to four hours. There are, however, no set rules and the breast-fed baby should be fed on demand whenever hungry. In general, a newborn will take between 8 and 12 feeds a day. Demand feeding will allow a natural pattern to emerge and as feeding becomes more established and the baby grows, feeds will become less frequent and more predictable. Although the baby should be fed on demand, it is important to remind the mother that a young baby should not sleep too long. A newborn who sleeps regularly for long periods at a time may need to be woken for feeds to promote the development of a feeding pattern and reduce the risk of dehydration.

A baby who continues to demand frequent feeds after the first week or so, may not be getting enough milk. This may be due to incorrect positioning or limiting time at the breast. The problem needs to be investigated and corrected otherwise feeding will not be successful.

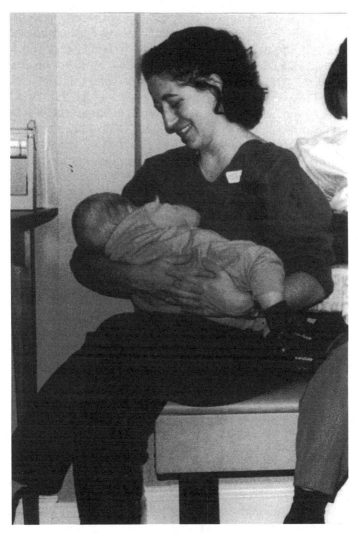

Fig. 2.2. Breast-feeding infant in 'belly to belly' position.

The length of time the baby feeds at the breast will also vary considerably. Some efficient feeders will be finished within ten minutes others may feed for twenty or thirty minutes. The baby should always be allowed to feed until satiated. There have been many rules about the length of time an infant should feed at each breast; however, it is now generally accepted that the infant should be allowed to feed fully from one breast before being offered the other. This enables the baby to take full advantage of the high fat, high calorie hind milk. The mother should be reassured that it does not matter if the baby does not take anything from the second breast at that feed, but she must alternate breasts at each feed. This will allow complete emptying of the breast and prevent engorgement.

Early weight loss   As has been said some early weight loss is inevitable in the breast-fed baby. Mothers should be prepared for this and reassured that no harm will result. The baby should be weighed regularly during the first week and only if the weight falls significantly is intervention necessary. In the past a weight loss up to 10% during the first ten days was considered acceptable and there appears, in the fullterm normal-sized infant to be no reason to depart from this rule of thumb. It is usual to expect that the baby will have regained birth weight somewhere between the tenth and fourteenth day. An adequate milk intake can usually be assumed if the infant is having between six and eight wet nappies daily and normal stools. Other reassuring signs include an alert and responsive baby, who is generally happy and content with good skin colour and some weight gain.

Some judgement is required. Occasionally a young baby may become dehydrated because of fever, diarrhoea, vomiting, or hyperventilation. From time to time an infant will lose weight at such a rapid rate that it is obvious that it will lose more than 10% of its weight. The administration of infant formula as a complement rather than supplement may be required to prevent malnutrition.

Complements and supplements   There are two alternative ways of providing a breast-fed infant with food other than breast milk.

Either the baby can be offered a bottle of infant formula immediately after a breast-feed (complementary feed) or it can be given a bottle independently of its breast-feeding pattern (supplementary feed).

It cannot be emphasized too strongly that the great majority of breast-fed babies do not require extra feeds and these should only be offered if there is a good reason to do so. There is evidence that giving babies formula during the period in which lactation is being established reduces the likelihood of success; there is a greatly increased chance that breast-feeding will stop altogether. It interferes with the cycle of hormonal stimulation which ensures maintenance and increase in milk secretion. We recommend avoiding bottle feeds of expressed breast milk or formula until the baby is around three weeks of age. Formula samples should not be given to a new mother as this has been shown to shorten the period for which they breast-feed. Also, it is not necessary to offer additional water or glucose water to the infant at any point; this may well interfere with the establishment of lactation. The occasional situation where extra feeds are justified is discussed elsewhere (pp. 24 and 127).

While all artificial feeds should be avoided during the early days, if for some reason extra intake is deemed necessary then complementary feeding is far preferable because it does not interfere with the natural rhythm of demand feeding.

Colostrum　　Colostrum is produced by the mammary gland during the first four to seven days after birth. This protein rich food has a specific amino acid composition, very high in arginine and tryptophan. It also has high levels of minerals, and vitamins particularly A as carotene, D, and B_{12}. The fat content—and therefore its energy content—is much lower than that of mature breast milk.

Much of the protein in colostrum consists of immunoglobulin (IgA) which may have a useful role to play in preventing infection and blocking early introduction of allergens through the gastrointestinal mucus membranes. Of the three important classes of immunoglobulins, IgG crosses the placenta so that the baby is effectively passively immunized by its mother against those antigens which evoke IgG antibodies, while IgM is produced by the fetus and therefore the newborn infant. Since IgA is not produced by the very young baby and does not cross the placenta colostrum, and to an extent mature breast milk, help to bridge the resulting antibody gap. Colostrum also contains living cells which are capable of releasing antibodies and other agents after ingestion. The presence of an antitrypsin factor prevents the digestion of much of the protein thus allowing the antibodies to survive in the gut during these early days.

Colostrum contains other anti-infective agents, including lysozyme which inhibits bacterial growth, and lactoferrin which binds iron in the intestine thus making it unavailable for bacterial growth. It also contains anti-inflammatory agents, hormones, growth factors, and enzymes.

The exact importance and roles of the antibodies, antibacterial agents, enzymes, and hormones in human milk is not yet fully understood but their presence appears to affect many aspects of growth and development of the infant and young child. The hormones present in human milk may be linked to brain development and general growth and development. There are many different enzymes present which assist with digestion, absorption, and transport of nutrients, some may also play a role in the preservation of components in the milk and prevent spoilage. As the baby matures, it becomes able to produce its own IgA which is secreted by gut epithelial cells onto the surface of the bowel where it exerts a protective effect.

Mature breast milk Frequent suckling by the infant during the first few days of life not only causes the amount of breast milk to increase but also results in its transformation into transitional (7–21 days) and then mature milk, with a gradual change in its nutritional composition. In fact, breast milk is never quite homogeneous and the initial part of the feed is always more similar to colostrum (the 'fore milk') than the milk secreted as the feed progresses (the 'hind milk'). The composition of so called mature milk is an averaging out of the transition which occurs within each feed. This 'average' product contains much less protein than colostrum and has a much higher fat and therefore energy content (Table 2.2). It still contains, albeit in lower concentrations, the antibodies, antibacterial agents, hormones, and enzymes present in colostrum but the total amount may not be reduced as the volume is greatly increased.

Table 2.2. Composition of mature human milk (per 100 ml)

Component	Human milk
Energy(kcal)	69
Protein(g)	1.3
Lactose(g)	7.2
Fat(g)	4.1
Vitamin(μg)	
A	60
D	0.04
E	0.34
K	0.21*
Thiamin	20
Riboflavin	30
Nicotinic Acid	200
B_{12}	Tr
B_6	10
Folate	5.0
Pantothenic Acid	250
Biotin	0.7
C(mg)	4.0
Sodium(mg)	15
Potassium(mg)	58
Chloride(mg)	42
Calcium(mg)	34
Phosphorus(mg)	15
Magnesium(mg)	3.0
Iron(mg)	0.07
Copper(mg)	0.04
Zinc(mg)	0.03
Iodine(μg)	7

*From Institute of Medicine (1991). *Nutrition during lactation*.

Adapted, with permission, from McCance, R. and Widdowson, E. (1995). *The composition of foods*, 5th edn. HMSO, London.

Human milk contains digestive enzymes, in particular lipase and amylase. These enable the young infant to absorb the fat and carbohydrate in the milk more effectively. Lipase is considered particularly important as infants depend upon a continuous supply of essential fatty acids and fat to maintain growth and development.

Mature human milk contains approximately 70 kcals 100 ml of which about 50% is derived from fat (Table 2.2). The remainder is provided by carbohydrate and any excess protein surplus to growth needs. The protein content of human milk is relatively low at 1.3 g/100 ml; however its absorption and bio-availability is high.

Lactose is the carbohydrate in milk. It is a disaccharide consisting of two monosaccharides, glucose and galactose. Before it can be absorbed, it is digested in the small bowel by the enzyme lactase. This enzyme is very vulnerable and defects in lactase are a relatively common cause of nutritional problems (see pp. 159 and 179).

Human milk contains all the vitamins, minerals, and trace elements known to be essential for the infant's needs provided that an adequate volume of milk is taken and that the mother's diet is satisfactory. It sometimes appears at first glance that the concentration of certain substances are low but two factors have to be taken into account; first that the 'bio-availability' (efficiency of absorption) of a mineral such as iron is very high in human milk and second there are a number of substances, i.e. copper, iron, and certain vitamins, that are built up during later pregnancy and which supplement the baby's supply during the first months of life. Premature babies and infants from some ethnic groups do not receive these stores and may be more likely to become deficient.

Drugs in breast milk

Most drugs taken by the mother during lactation either do not harm the baby or pass into breast milk in such low concentrations that they are harmless. Nevertheless care should be taken regarding drugs prescribed to the lactating mother. The British National Formulary carries an excellent and authoritative review of the relative risks of drugs which may pass into breast milk. We have given some commonly prescribed drugs which are known to be safe and have listed some of those which are 'best avoided' (Table 2.3). However, since the list of drugs and their side-effects is long and growing it is important always to consult

Table 2.3. Common drugs and breast-feeding mothers

Drug	Comments/risk to infant
Amphetamines	Significant amount in milk. Avoid
Anticoagulants (oral), including phenindione	Risk of haemorrhage increased by vitamin K deficiency. Avoid
Warfarin	Appears safe
Antidepressants (tricyclics)	Amount of tricyclic antidepressants (including related drugs such as mianserin and trazodone) too small to be harmful; manufacturers advise avoidance; accumulation of doxepin metabolite may cause sedation and respiratory depression
Aspirin	Avoid—possible risk of Reye's syndrome; impaired platelet function and hypoprothrombinaemia if vitamin K stores low
Barbiturates	Avoid; large doses may produce drowsiness
Beta-blockers	Amount excreted in milk small; monitor infant for possible toxicity due to beta-blockade
Carbamezepine	Amount probably too small to be harmful, severe skin reaction has been reported
Carbimazole	Use lowest effective dose as amount in milk may affect neonatal thyroid function
Codeine	Secreted in breast milk in very small amounts unlikely to be harmful
Contraceptives (oral—combination)	Avoid until after weaning or six months after birth as have adverse effect on lactation
Progesterone-only	Do not affect lactation can be started three weeks after birth

Table 2.3. (*continued*)

Drug	Comments/risk to infant
Corticosteroids	Continuous therapy with high doses (>10 mg prednisolone daily) could affect infant's adrenal function; monitor carefully
Ibuprofen	Amount too small to be harmful, but some manufacturers recommend avoid
Lithium salts	Monitor infant for possible intoxication; low incidence of adverse effects but increased by continuous ingestion; good control of maternal plasma levels minimizes risk
Morphine	Therapeutic doses unlikely to affect infant; withdrawal symptoms in infants of dependent mothers; breast-feeding therefore contraindicated
Paracetamol	Amount too small to be harmful
Penecillins	Trace amounts in breast milk; not generally harmful
Phenobarbitone	Avoid when possible; drowsiness may occur but risk probably small
Phenytoin	Small amount excreted in milk; manufacturer advises avoid
Tetracyclines	Avoid

Note: Many drugs are excreted in breast milk and pose a possible threat to the infant of a breast-feeding mother. The above short list refers to those which are perhaps most commonly a cause for concern. A more comprehensive list can be found as an Appendix in the *British National Formulary*.

the Formulary before prescribing or taking a drug not mentioned here.

Alcohol is excreted in breast milk and will produce drowsiness in the infant if taken in large amounts. It is recommended that the breast-feeding mother avoids alcohol completely; however, an occasional glass of wine or beer taken with food is unlikely to have adverse effects. It is also advisable to avoid large amounts of caffeine containing beverages such as coffee.

Environmental pollution is another concern. Babies both artificially fed and breast-fed ingest small quantities of pesticide residues although these levels may have fallen recently. There is no evidence that present levels are harmful, but this is an area where there is no room for complacency and the addition of non-biodegradable or slowly degradable residues to the environment should be actively resisted. The Chernobyl disaster has also raised concern about radioactivity in milk. There is evidence that breast-fed babies suffered less ingestion of substances such as radioactive iodine than did formula-fed infants. During periods where there is a risk of radioactive contamination babies should be breast-fed as long as possible.

Although water is generally microbiologically safe in Britain, in certain agricultural areas, nitrate run-off from fertilizers may enter the water supply and can pose a danger, for example in some drought conditions. Lead may be present in higher than acceptable concentrations if the supply pipes are made of lead and the water is very soft.

Fluoride in water remains an emotive issue. It poses no threat to either the breast- or bottle-fed infant. Fluoridation of water supplies where the levels are below average is harmless and should be advocated as a sensible preventive measure. There is little doubt that it will reduce the prevalence of dental caries, which although falling is still too high.

Maternal diet during pregnancy and lactation

Good nutrition and a well-balanced diet are important from before conception, during pregnancy and during lactation, both for the well-being of the mother and the child. Little is known about the effects of pre-conceptual nutrition on the development of the fetus but a varied diet as recommended in the National Food Guide (see Chapter 5) is desirable with adequate energy intake and a balance of all nutrients. There is now strong evidence that intake of folic acid at conception and during the first trimester of pregnancy is important in preventing certain congenital anomalies, particularly spina bifida and other neural tube defects. Women likely to become pregnant should ensure that their diet contains adequate amounts of folate (400 μg daily). Table 2.4 gives some examples of foods high in folic acid, in addition foods fortified with folic acid should be included. Vitamin

Table 2.4. Foods high in folic acid

Food	Folic Acid content per serving(μg)
Orange 1 whole	30
Orange juice 150 ml (5 oz) glass	30
Clementines 2 whole	30
Banana 1 medium	16
Brussels sprouts*	100
Spinach*	80
Broccoli*	58
Spring greens*	60
Curly kale*	80
Peas*	40
Baked beans 100 g (3½ oz)	22
Peanuts 30 g (1 oz)	15
Fortified breakfast cereals 30 g (1 oz)	75
e.g. Rice Krispies, Cornflakes, Bran Flakes	
granary bread** 2 slices	50

*Vegetables should be very lightly cooked to avoid destroying the folate. Calculations based on cooked, fresh vegetables, average serving sizes of approximately 90 g (3–3½ oz).
**Also look for other fortified breads, they may contain more folate.

supplements containing 400 μg folic acid are recommended if there is any doubt about the content of the diet (there is some evidence that consumption of folate fortified foods and folate supplements are better at improving folate status than folate rich foods). Women who have previously had a child with a neural tube defect are recommended to consume even higher amounts of folate preconceptually and during pregnancy.

Alcohol should be either avoided entirely or reduced to a minimal intake. The recommended allowance for a non-pregnant women is not more than two glasses of wine or its equivalent per day and during pregnancy the intake should be considerably less than this. Alcoholism is associated with a pattern of congenital abnormalities so characteristic that it is called the fetal-alcohol syndrome.

Since many women will not realize that they are pregnant for several weeks, pre-conceptual diet will necessarily be the same for the early part of pregnancy.

During the second and third trimesters of pregnancy rapid growth of the fetus imposes increased nutritional demands on the mother. The exact requirements vary with each individual and the reference nutrient intakes (RNIs; see Table 2.5) can be used as a general guide. Extra energy is required because of the needs of the growing fetus and also because during pregnancy there is an increase in maternal fat stores which are subsequently available for lactation. However as many women reduce their activity and therfore energy expenditure they do not need to increase their energy intake dramatically. It is calculated that a 10% increase is required when physical activity remains the

Table 2.5. Reference nutrient intakes of selected nutrients for pregnant and lactating women

Nutrient	Pregnancy	Lactation 0–4 months	Lactation 4+ months
Energy (EAR) (kcal)	+ 200*	+ 450–570**	+ 570–240**
Protein(g)	+ 6*	+ 11*	+ 8*
Thiamin(mg)	+ 0.1 (last trimester)	+ 0.2*	+ 0.2*
Riboflavin(mg)	+ 0.3*	+ 0.5*	+ 0.5*
Folate(μg)	+ 100*	+ 60*	+ 60*
Vitamin C(mg)	+ 10*	+ 30*	+ 30*
Vitamin A(μg)	+ 100*	+ 350*	+ 350*
Vitamin D(μg)	10	10	10
Calcium(mmol)	no increment	+ 14.3*	+ 14.3*
Iron(μg)	no increment	no increment	no increment

EAR: estimated average requirement.

*add to adult requirement.
**varies according to amount of milk produced/ exclusive or partial breast-feeds/ weaning.

(Adapted from: Department of Health (1991). Report on health and social subjects. *Dietary reference values for food, energy and nutrients for the United Kingdom*. Report No. 41. HMSO, UK).

same. The best guide is to base energy needs on the rate of weight gain.

Although protein requirement is high, most average British diets provide more than adequate amounts. Protein is particularly important during the last 8–9 weeks as the fetus lays down about two thirds of its total body nitrogen and tissue protein during this period.

During the last trimester the fetus will also lay down stores of vitamins and minerals which are important during the early months of post-uterine life. This is illustrated by the deficiency states which can occur in preterm babies who do not have these reserves. Therefore the diet of the mother should contain enough vitamins and minerals to meet this increased need. In certain groups who are specially at risk of dietary deficiency, vitamin supplementation is desirable, for example vitamin D in Asian women. Women who smoke, an undesirable habit during pregnancy for many reasons, may need extra vitamin C due to the reduced absorption of ascorbic acid. It is important to note that excessive supplementation can also be dangerous, for example high intakes of vitamin A (over 3000 μg or 10 000 IU/day), have been linked to birth defects. Pregnant women should therefore be advised to avoid taking supplements containing vitamin A and not to eat liver or liver products because of their very high content of this vitamin.

Of minerals, iron, calcium, and copper demands are all increased, partly because they are incorporated in fetal tissues and partly in the case of iron and copper because they are stored in the liver. Additionally the expansion of the number of red blood cells in the mother increases the demand for iron. In women with good iron reserves, this increased demand is met by including high iron foods such as kidney, red meat, pulses, fortified cereals, and green leaf vegetables. This should be accompanied by foods containing nutrients which aid the absorption of iron such as vitamin C and folate.

Calcium intake can be achieved provided the diet contains sufficient vitamin D or there is adequate exposure to sunlight. High-fibre diets in themselves desirable during pregnancy may reduce absorption of calcium. It is thus essential that at least the usual recommendation of 700–800 mg of calcium is consumed daily. This can be met by including foods rich in calcium, such as milk, cheese, yoghurt, and tinned fish in the diet (Table 2.6). The alternative is to provide calcium as a supplement.

The maternal diet during lactation should provide increased quantities of foods to meet increased nutritional requirements. A normal and varied diet based on healthy eating principles as outlined in the *National Food Guide* (see Chapter 5) is to be recommended. Some specific nutrients are needed in much larger amounts during lactation, for example calcium requirements are increased from about 800 mg to 1350 mg. There is also an increased requirement for vitamins A, D, and C. If the extra energy required is met from foods which contain a proper balance of nutrients supplementation is not usually necessary.

Table 2.6. Some examples of food rich in calcium

Food	Portion size providing approximately 250 mg calcium
Milk	200 ml (⅓ pint)
Cheese	30 g (1 oz)
Yoghurt—plain	125 g (1–1½ cartons)
—fruit	150 g (1–1½ cartons)
Fromage frais	280 g (10 oz)
Sardines (tinned)	60 g (2 oz)
Almonds	100 g (3½ oz)
Tofu (calcium fortified)	60 g (2 oz)
Fortified soya milk	300 ml (½ pint)
	Portion size providing approximately 50 mg calcium
Salmon (tinned)	60 g (2 oz)
Raisins	100 g (3½ oz)
Sultanas	90 g (3 oz)
Sunflower seeds	50 g (2 oz)

Fluid intake during lactation will in effect be maintained by the normal thirst mechanisms and will increase.

Maternal diet has little effect on the total amount of nutrients in breast milk; however, the proportion of different fatty acids does vary with maternal dietary intake. The vitamin content is also a reflection of maternal intake and stores and could be depleted in the breast milk if the mother had a chronically low intake.

Sometimes substances other than drugs present in food may have an untoward effect on the baby. It is claimed that very spicy foods or orange juice can produce loose stools. While such effects are not harmful it may be sensible to avoid offending foods if they cause concern, provided this does not have an effect on overall dietary intake. Occasionally, allergens may reach the baby in the breast milk and if there is good evidence that the baby is reacting to them, then the offending food should be avoided. Care should be taken to ensure that the problem is genuinely due to the food and not to some other cause.

Supplementary vitamins

Whether breast-fed babies should receive supplementary vitamins is controversial. The official recommendation is that vitamins, A, D, and C should be given to full term, breast-fed infants from six months of age unless the mother's diet is known to be nutritionally adequate. The difficulty in this recommendation is establishing that the diet is nutritionally adequate, something that can only be ensured by a detailed dietary history, and for this reason some health professionals recommend vitamin supplements from one month of age. A vitamin K supplement of 1.0 mg should be given to all infants at birth in order to prevent haemorrhagic disease of the newborn. If this is given by intramuscular injection no further dose is required; if given by mouth, breast-fed infants should receive repeat doses at one and four weeks of age.

The standard vitamin supplement available through health clinics contains adequate levels of vitamins, A, D, and C (Table 2.7). If the mother is insistent that she does not wish to give the baby a vitamin supplement and it is suspected that her diet may not be

Table 2.7. Welfare vitamins

Five drops contain:	
Vitamin A	200 μg
Vitamin D	7 μg
Vitamin C	20 mg

Recommended for all children up to the age of five years.

adequate, then a full dietary assessment by a qualified dietitian is necessary.

How long should mothers breast-feed?

Mothers should be encouraged to breast-feed their babies as long as possible and at least until the baby is weaned onto solids (6–9 months), but there is no reason why it should not continue thereafter for as long as is mutually satisfying for mother and infant. Breast milk will provide adequate nutrition for all fully breast-fed babies until 5–6 months of age. Thereafter in a significant proportion of infants weight gain will slacken, hence the need for the introduction of solids at this stage.

Bottle-feeding

In developed countries, bottle-feeding is a generally safe and a satisfactory alternative to breast-feeding provided that an approved infant formula is used. These formulas attempt to mimic as far as possible the composition of mature human milk but they cannot mirror its complex immunological, hormonal, and enzyme content. Nor do they necessarily have similar amino acid or fatty acid composition. Some formulas have recently added long-chain polyunsaturated fatty acids (LCPs). These are not normally present in infant formula, but are present in breast milk and thought to be essential for premature infants. Some recent research has indicated that these may be necessary for fullterm infants. LCPs are known to be important in the structural lipids of the developing brain, and play an important functional role in the central nervous system. At this time there is no official ruling on the addition of LCPs to infant formula.

Despite these qualifications, if a mother chooses to bottle-feed her baby she can rest assured that there are available prefectly adequate feeds from a nutritional point of view. The guidelines for what constitutes an infant formula are laid down by the UK Government in line with European Community and World Health Organisation regulations.

Most infant formulas are based on cows' milk and fall into two main categories, whey-based and casein-based. Casein-based formulas are essentially diluted cows' milk to which nutrients are added but the ratio of casein to whey protein is similar to that of cows' milk. Whey-based formulas are more highly modified and have whey protein added so that the casein to whey ratio is more like that of human milk. Since whey protein contains more essential amino acids than casein it is possible to achieve lower protein levels in whey-based formulas. Each baby food manufacturer tends to produce one whey-based and one casein-based formula (Table 2.8). Whey-based formulas most closely resemble human milk in protein and mineral content.

The carbohydrate present in most infant formulas is lactose as in cows' milk and human milk but other carbohydrates such as maltodextrin are permitted. All these formulas have a similar nutritional content and are all satisfactory infant feeds. Any other milk-based product which does not meet the criterion of a baby food is considered unsuitable as an infant formula. These include unmodified cows' milk, evaporated milk, goats' milk, sheeps' milk, and unmodified soya 'milk'.

Bottle-fed infants should be demand fed in much the same way as breast-fed infants, enabling them to regulate their own volume of intake. An average intake of 150–200 ml/kg/day is a useful guide-line but it is important to remember that babies differ greatly in their requirements. From about the age of six weeks babies develop an internal sensor which enables them to control their caloric intake, provided the feed is made up to the correct caloric density (not too concentrated or too dilute).

The position in which the baby is bottle-fed is also important. The baby should be held in a supportive, semi-upright, position,

Table 2.8. Selected nutrient composition of infant formulas, follow-on formulas, and cows' milk

(A) Whey-based infant formulas

Nutrient (per 100 ml)	Boots Formula 1	C&G Premium	Farley's First Milk	Milupa Aptamil*	SMA Gold
Energy (kcal)	67	66	68	67	67
Protein (g)	1.5	1.4	1.4	1.5	1.5
Casein (%)	40	40	39	40	40
Whey (%)	60	60	61	60	60
Fat (g)	3.5	3.6	3.8	3.6	3.6
Carbohydrate (g)	7.4	7.1	7.0	7.2	7.2
Sodium (mg)	19	17.8	17	23	16
Potassium (mg)	46	66.7	57	82	65
Calcium (mg)	39	53.3	39	66	46
Iron (mg)	0.8	0.5	0.6	0.7	0.8
Thiamin (µg)	65	38	42	40	100
Riboflavin (µg)	78	110	55	50	150
Folate (µg)	3.9	10	3.4	10	8.0
Vitamin C (mg)	9.8	7.6	6.9	8	9.0
Vitamin A (µg)	84	76.2	100	60	75
Vitamin D (µg)	1.0	1.1	1.0	1.0	1.1

*contains added long chain polyunsaturated fatty acids (LCPs).

(B) Casein-based infant formulas

Nutrient (per 100 ml)	Boots Formula 2	C&G Plus	Farley's Second milk	Milupa Milumil	SMA White
Energy (kcal)	68	66	66	68	67
Protein (g)	1.6	1.7	1.7	1.9	1.6
Casein (%)	80	80	77	80	80
Whey (%)	20	20	23	20	20
Fat (g)	3.6	3.4	2.9	3.1	3.6
Carbohydrate (g)	7.2	7.2	8.3	8.1	7.0
Sodium (mg)	22	25	25	26	22
Potassium (mg)	73	90	86	98	80
Calcium (mg)	59	80	61	88	56
Iron (mg)	0.8	0.5	0.7	0.7	0.8
Thiamin (µg)	50	40	39	40	100
Riboflavin (µg)	60	100	53	60	150
Folate (µg)	7	10	3.3	11	8.0
Vitamin C (mg)	8	8	6.6	8.0	9.0
Vitamin A (µg)	70	80	97	63	75
Vitamin D (µg)	1.0	1.1	1.0	1.1	1.1

(C) Follow-on formulas and cow's milk

Nutrient (per 100 ml)	Whole Cow's Milk	Boots Follow-on Milk	C & G Step-up	Farley's Follow-on Milk	Milupa Forward	SMA Progress
Energy (Kcal)	68	65	70	68	74	67
Protein (g)	3.2	2.2	1.8	2.1	2.1	2.2
Fat (g)	4.0	3.4	3.8	3.1	3.3	3.0
Carbohydrate (g)	4.7	6.4	7.2	8.0	9.0	7.8
Sodium (mg)	57	29	23	31	34	33
Potassium (mg)	144	97	86	91	115	107
Calcium (mg)	119	69	88	72	87	90
Iron (mg)	0.05	1.3	1.3	1.2	1.2	1.3
Thiamin (μg)	40	42	40	40	40	100
Riboflavin (μg)	180	63	100	150	150	150
Folate (μg)	6.0	3.9	11.0	7.0	11.0	8.0
Vitamin C (mg)	1.0	6.8	8.0	10	9.0	9.0
Vitamin A (μg)	58	110	60	80	62	75
Vitamin D (μg)	0.03	1.3	1.8	1.1	1.0	1.2

which encourages eye contact and bonding with the caregiver (see Chapter 7, Fig. 7.2).

The total volume of feed may be divided in 6, 7, or 8 feeds as appropriate. The exact timing and number of feeds is usually dictated by the individual infant, young babies usually demanding 7–8 feeds per day. The number of feeds per day falls gradually as the infant becomes larger. The first feed to be dropped is usually the night feed which is no longer necessary after four months of age. The baby then gradually goes longer before demanding to be fed so that at about two months many infants are feeding approximately every four hours without a night feed. They thus obtain their full requirement from about 5–6 feeds per day. If a baby is offered too few feeds for its age or maturity it may not be able to cope with the increased feed volume needed to maintain nutrition. The average number of feeds and volumes of feeds at different ages is summarized in Table 2.9. It should be emphasized that these are averages and that babies show considerable individual variations in their needs.

The formulas should be mixed exactly according to the manufacturer's instructions. In the UK this is standardized to 1 level scoop of formula powder to 30 ml (1 fluid ounce) of water. The water should be boiled and allowed to cool slightly before mixing. Only the standard scoop provided should be used. Dramatic alterations in the concentration of the formula may result from compression of the powder in the scoop or by using heaped

Table 2.9. Average number and volume of feeds at different ages

Approximate age	Approximate feed volume (single feed)	Number of feeds
1–2 weeks	50–70 ml	7–8
2–6 weeks	75–110 ml	6–7
2 months	110–180 ml	5–6
3 months	170–220 ml	5
6 months*	220–240 ml	4

These figures are merely for guidance. Many babies will vary the volume ingested from day-to-day and from feed-to-feed.
*Weaning foods will also contribute to nutrient intake at this age.

scoops. Overconcentration of the feed may lead to hyperna-traemia (raised serum sodium) with dehydration and this can lead to severe brain damage or death. Much of this danger has been reduced since the introduction of highly modified infant formula but it has not been entirely eliminated. It is possible that inappropriate caloric density may 'confuse' the internal sensor mechanism and cause overfeeding and subsequent obesity (see Chapters 7 and 10). Over dilute feeds may lead to excessive volumes being ingested in order to meet caloric requirement and this can cause vomiting and hyponatraemia. Failure to thrive and malnutrition may ensue because the capacity of the young infant's stomach cannot cope with the much larger volumes of feed required to maintain nutrition.

Partly because bottle-fed babies do not have the degree of immunological protection of breast-fed babies and partly because of the potential risk of contamination, hygiene during the preparation of feeds is of the utmost importance. All feeding equipment and any utensils used during the mixing of the feed must be sterilized. The simplest and most widely used method of sterilization are proprietary sterilizing agents such as Milton, Boots, or Maws. These usually contain hypochlorite solution and equipment should be immersed for the specified period.

Feeds can be mixed for a full 24-hour period provided they are stored in a refrigerator. The feed should be removed immediately prior to feeding and warmed to at least room temperature before feeding the baby. Prolonged standing of the feed in a warm environment such as a bottle warmer, near a fire, or on a radiator will create the ideal medium for bacterial growth and should be actively discouraged. Once the feed has been warmed for use it should not be returned to the refrigerator for re-use. Using the microwave oven to warm feeds in the bottle is a dangerous practice because milk in the centre of the bottle may be very hot, and if not noticed may scald the baby.

Supplementary vitamins

Bottle-fed babies generally receive adequate amounts of vitamins and minerals from infant formula. At six months of age it is recommended that they are given the welfare vitamin drops (see Table 2.7) and that these are continued untill five years of age in all children.

Drinks

Extra drinks of fruit juice or boiled water should not generally be encouraged for either breast-fed or bottle-fed babies particularly during the first two weeks of life as they will interfere with the establishment of feeding. It is not usually necessary to give breast-fed infants any drinks at all.

If a bottle-fed infant is thirsty or cries between feeds particularly in hot weather, drinks of cool boiled water should be offered. Fruit juices should not be offered before three months and are not necessary until after weaning. All fruit juices and baby drinks contain glucose or fructose. These, although less harmful than sucrose, can cause dental caries. They should be used very infrequently and well diluted with water, we would recommend at least three parts water to one part juice. Dummies and comforters should never be dipped in concentrated fruit juice.

Introduction of cows' milk

Breast milk or infant formula should be the sole liquid feed until at least six months of age. It is now recommended that this should be continued until the child is one year old, or a follow-up milk may be used after six months. Cow's milk is not recommended until the baby is one year old as it has a high solute load, is too low in some vitamins and minerals, notably iron, which becomes important from about six months when antenatal stores have been consumed. Also, cows' milk is more likely to be contaminated by bacteria than feeds prepared from formulas.

The main difference between follow-up milks and infant formulas is their higher protein and sodium content making them unsuitable for infants under six months of age (Table 2.8). In our opinion follow-up milks are expensive and have no real advantage over continued breast-feeding or formula during the second six months and seem to introduce an unnecessary complication. The main argument in their favour is the fact that they are iron fortified giving them an advantage over cows' milk which is not recommended anyway. Infant formula is also iron fortified and can also be used in the second sixth months of life. Iron deficiency anaemia is a problem in this age group and a source of dietary iron must be provided, usually from infant formula and solid foods such as baby cereal fortified with iron. Follow-up formulas may have a role in preventing iron deficiency anaemia in those infants who will not take infant formula. Skimmed milk and semi-skimmed milks are not suitable for babies under two years of age (see Chapter 5).

Feeding weanlings

Weaning is the process which begins when breast- or bottle-feeding starts to be replaced by a mixed diet. The term weaning means to cease to be suckled. Weaning onto solid food should be a gradual process over several weeks and months starting somewhere between four and six months of age. The exact time will be dictated by the individual infant and mother.

Weaning is necessary when breast milk or infant formula are no longer able to provide adequate nutrition for the growing infant. It also plays an important role in the development of chewing and there appears to be a fairly critical time for the introduction of solids by six months to ensure normal chewing development and possibly later speech development. Babies may also be less receptive to new tastes after six months of age.

Weaning is commenced with the introduction of a small quantity of a smooth bland gluten-free cereal or puréed fruit without added sugar. Initially offer:

- 1–2 teaspoons then gradually increase
- start at one feed before or after the breast- or bottle-feed
- use a strong plastic weaning spoon
- never add solids to the bottle
- place only a small quantity of food on the spoon.

Many babies will refuse the first offer of solids and it is important to emphasize the need to persevere but under no circumstances must the baby be force-fed. If the baby is upset by the first attempt it should immediately be breast- or bottle-fed and another attempt made later. Sometimes solids may be offered during the course of a breast- or bottle-feed when the baby, having overcome his initial hunger may show more curiosity about the new food. Mothers should be aware of basic hygiene, for example the need to wash hands before preparing the food and feeding it to the baby and the need to keep utensils clean and that all equipment used for preparing weaning foods can be sterilized in a similar way to feeding bottles.

Following the first introduction to solids, a gradual increase in the quantity, number of solid feeds, and the variety of foods offered should take place. The exact pace will to some extent be dictated by the baby and the confidence of the mother. There are a wide range of proprietary weaning foods available either as ready to feed or in a dried form requiring the addition of water or milk. Both savoury and sweet flavours should be given and variety is important in developing the baby's sense of taste and smell. Salt and sugar should never be added to food. Homemade weaning foods can easily be prepared using fresh foods from normal family meals provided that no salt or sugar have been added. They can be brought to the correct consistency using a baby mouli, sieve, food-processor, or liquidizer. Their advantage is that they are cheaper than proprietary foods but can be less convenient and less nutrient dense. The amount of milk taken will gradually fall as the solid food intake rises. The changes in feeding which occur during weaning are illustrated by the sample menus in Fig. 2.3.

By the age of six months babies may be ready to start some finger feeding. They should be offered a small finger of toast, a rusk, or a small piece of fruit and allowed to experiment with it. The baby should not be left alone with these but should be encouraged to feed himself, however messy the outcome. A gradual introduction of more solid foods and lumpy foods will take place until by one year the child will be taking a variety of solid foods. In the allergic child or where there is a strong family history of allergy, precautions to avoid highly allergic foods until after 1 year of age may be appropriate (see Chapter 9).

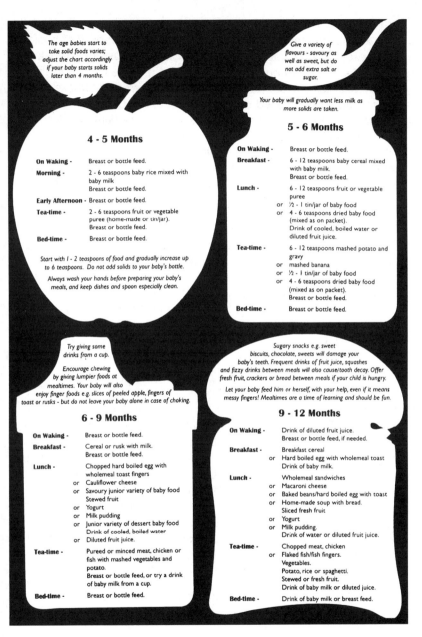

Fig. 2.3. Weaning stages. Reproduced with permission, British Dietetic Association, Paediatric Group.

From about 6 months liquids can be offered from a cup (see Fig. 2.3). Emphasis should be placed on the desirability of avoiding sweet biscuits, chocolates, and sweets because of the risk of dental caries. Frequent drinks of fruit juice, squashes, and fizzy drinks are also deleterious to the teeth. Fresh fruit, crackers, or bread should be offered if the baby is hungry between meals. It is important to note that certain snack foods particularly peanuts pose a choking hazard and should be avoided completely.

At one year of age cows' milk can be introduced as a drink. Whole milk should always be recommended and at least one pint per day is necessary to ensure adequate nutrition in an average child in an average family.

Weaning the breast-fed baby

There are no differences in principle between breast-fed and bottle-fed weanlings. From about five months it becomes increasingly unlikely that breast milk alone will meet the needs of the infant and solids should be gradually introduced. It is not necessary to introduce any infant formula during the weaning process and the mother should be encouraged to continue to breast-feed (see Fig. 2.3).

Feeding the preterm infant

Prospects for the preterm infant have steadily improved over the past two decades so that even infants born as early as 25 weeks gestation now have around a 50% survival rate. The provision of effective nutritional support for this vulnerable group has become an area of increasing importance. Optimum nutrition should lead to normal growth and development uncomplicated by infection or metabolic disturbance. Formula feeds for preterm infants are continually being refined and the ideal composition is unknown. What is clear, however, is that use of term formula is inappropriate since it clearly lacks sufficient nutrients and that breast milk alone may not be sufficient for these infants.

Preterm infant formula

Formula feeds for the preterm infant have been modified to include more energy, protein, and minerals (Table 2.10). Impressive trials conducted by Dr. Alan Lucas and colleagues in the 1980s have shown that infants born prematurely and fed preterm rather than term formula not only grow faster but make better developmental progress.

These findings are almost certainly attributable to the differences in nutrient intake. However, when donor breast milk and preterm formula were compared there was little difference in subsequent development scores at eighteen months of age despite this being the most extreme nutritional contrast investigated. This suggests that there is something about breast milk which confers neurodevelopmental advantage. Data from these studies showed that even at 7.5 years of age, children of mothers who decided to express their breast milk had significant developmental advantages.

Breast milk

There are both advantages and disadvantages in the use of breast milk for preterm infants. Drip-milk collected from the non-suckling breast by nursing mothers in the community has provided a source of human milk for many neonatal units in the past.

Table 2.10. Selected nutrient content of feeds for preterm infants

Nutrient (per 100 ml)	Preterm formula	Term formula	Mother's expressed breast milk*	Banked donor breast milk*
Protein(g)	2.0	1.5	1.5	1.1
Fat(g)	4.9	3.8	3.0	1.7
Carbohydrate(g)	7.0	7.0	7.0	7.1
Energy(kcal)	80	68	62	46
Sodium(mg)	45	19	23	16
Calcium(mg)	70	35	35	35
Phosphorus(mg)	35	29	15	15

*Mean values from analysis of pooled samples; from Morely and Lucas (unpublished).

Whilst mother's milk is ideal for the term newborn, increasing doubts have been expressed regarding its appropriateness for the preterm infant.

Disadvantages of mother's milk for the preterm infant include:

- low fat, sodium, and mineral content of donor milk
- expressed milk is heterogeneous in composition
- poor growth rates compared with preterm formula feeding
- potential vector for viral transmission (e.g. Hepatitis B, HIV)
- pasteurization destroys antimicrobiological properties
- milk banking is labour intensive.

On the positive side breast milk appears to contain factors which promote brain growth and development. Likely candidates are long-chain fatty acids, notably docosa-hexaenoic and arachidonic acids which are found in abundance in the brain and retina. These substances are now being introduced into formula milks, although the long-term clinical benefits of this have yet to be demonstrated. Despite the fact that many studies have indicated breast-feeding may promote cognitive development, recent epidemiological work has suggested that any link between type of feeding in early life with later intelligence is most likely to be explained by the child's social environment. This remains a controversial topic, but the rapid growth and development of the preterm brain may make it particularly susceptible to nutritional influences.

Another important finding from recent studies was an apparent protective effect of breast milk against necrotizing enterocolitis (NEC). This is a major cause of morbidity and mortality amongst preterm infants, affecting around 8% of those less than 1500 g birth weight. It has been estimated that if all babies could be given mother's milk, the impact on NEC would be such that there would be 500 fewer cases in the UK each year with 100 fewer deaths.

Breast milk from a mother who has just given birth to a preterm infant differs in composition from that of a mother with a term infant. During the first few days of lactation preterm milk has a higher concentration of protein, sodium, and chloride as if it were especially adapted to the needs of a premature infant.

The advantages of mother's milk for the preterm infant can be summarized as follows:

- expressing mother is directly involved in care of child, aids bonding
- neurodevelopmental advantage despite nutritional 'inadequacy' (?related to content of long-chain fatty acids)
- protective against necrotizing enterocolitis (even when pasteurized).

These benefits of breast milk have elaborated after a steady decline in use of donor milk, only one third of regional neonatal units in the UK now have access to banked milk. This has lead to renewed efforts to support mothers who wish to express their milk, coupled with the evaluation of cup-feeding techniques as an alternative to nasogastric tube feeds, in the hope that this might increase the proportion of premature infants going home breast-fed. At the same time, supplements to breast milk have become available which, when added, increase the sodium, mineral, and carbohydrate content of the feed, making it more like a preterm formula. Although these supplements have been shown to increase weight gain, only short-term studies have so far been conducted. In view of this it is perhaps of some concern that their use has become standard practice in many neonatal units.

Feeding premature infants in the community

For the bottle-fed infant, preterm formula milk is usually discontinued by the time of discharge home and a term formula is substituted. The timing of this change varies between different centres, some using a post-conceptional age of 34 weeks, others a weight cut-off of 1.8 or 2.0 kg, while still others simply choose the time of discharge. Many infants will be sent home from hospital little more than half the weight of a term infant, often with weight and length below the third centile. Given the demands of catch-up growth, a term formula from the time of discharge may not adequately meet the nutritional needs of some infants. Such concerns have led to the development of so-called premature infant follow-on milks (e.g. Farley's Premcare,

Cow and Gate Nutriprem 2). These provide additional energy, protein, and minerals compared with a standard term formula and are intermediate in composition between a term and preterm formula. There is some evidence that babies given this type of preterm formula have improved bone mineralization and do gain weight and length more quickly than those receiving term formula; however, the long-term benefits of this improved weight gain are uncertain, and head growth (and therefore brain growth) does not seem to be enhanced. Until more evidence supporting the use of premature follow-on formulas is available, they should be used with caution under the supervision of a paediatrician and paediatric dietitian.

Preterm infants should routinely receive vitamin supplements and most (although not all) units usually prescribe iron. Although weaning does not have to begin until the infant is 4–6 months corrected age (corrected age = time since birth [i.e. 'chronological age'] less weeks of prematurity), there are some babies who seem to become dissatisfied with milk feeds long before this time. It seems reasonable to allow weaning in these infants when weight has reached 5 kg, the extrusion reflex is lost (the tongue no longer automatically pushes food out), and the child is able to eat from a spoon. Particular attention should be paid to providing appropriate energy and nutrient dense foods. Some of these infants develop feeding difficulties or are fussy eaters and because of their special nutritional needs should be referred to a paediatric dietitian.

Further reading

Committee on Medical Aspects of Food Policy (1994). *Weaning and the weaning diet*. Report on Health and Social Subjects, No. 45. HMSO, London.

Davies, D.P. (1995). Human milk: a sacred cow? A quest for optimum nutrition for pre-term babies. In *Nutrition in child health* (ed. D.P. Davies), pp. 53–65. Royal College of Physicians of London, London.

Department for Health and Social Security (1988). *Present day practices in infant feeding*. Report on health and social subjects, No. 32, (Third Report). HMSO, London.

Meah, S. (1996). Breast-milk feeding the preterm neonate. *Seminars in Neonatology*, **1**, 3–10.

Morley, R. and Lucas, A. (1995). The influence of early diet on outcome in pre-term infants. In *Nutrition in child health* (ed. D.P. Davies), pp. 67–75. Royal College of Physicians of London, London.

Wald, N.J. and Bower, C. (1995). Folic acid and the prevention of neural tube defects: a population strategy is needed. *British Medical Journal*, **310**, 1019–1120.

Zipursky, A. (1996). Vitamin K at birth. *British Medical Journal*, **7051**, (313), 179–180.

3

The preschoolchild

The preschool years represent a time of changing nutritional needs, from the totally dependent infant whose diet consists primarily of milk to an independent feeder who is consuming a mixed diet based on normal family foods. There are few studies of the dietary habits of preschoolchildren and until recently no major surveys of British children. The *National diet and nutrition survey* (HMSO 1995) on the food habits of British children between the ages of 1½ and 4½ years now provides us with insight into what young children are eating and future studies are planned. There are, however, reference nutrient intake (RNI) values for many nutrients (Table 3.1). In recent years, studies of the nutrient intakes of young children in Britain, the United States, and other countries have seen a downward trend in fat intakes. Preschoolchildren now appear to be consuming about 34%–36% of their energy from fat, although there may be a trend for this to increase as the child gets older. Since the 1960s, the energy intake of British preschoolchildren has been decreasing. This would appear to be a consequence of lower activity levels and heated homes, which have led to decreased energy needs. In the United States this trend has not been the same and energy intakes seem to have remained constant, with a larger

Table 3.1. Reference nutrient intakes of selected nutrients for preschoolchildren

Nutrient	1–3 years		4–6 years	
Energy (EAR)	male	female	male	female
(kcal)	1230	1165	1715	1545
Protein (g)	14.5		19.7	
Thiamin (mg)	0.5		0.7	
Riboflavin (mg)	0.6		0.8	
Folate (μg)	70		100	
Vitamin C (mg)	30		30	
Vitamin A (μg)	400		400	
Vitamin D (μg)	7		–	
Calcium (mmol)	8.8 (350 mg)		11.3 (450 mg)	
Iron (μg)	120 (6.9 mg)		110 (6.1 mg)	

EAR: estimated average requirement.

(Adapted from: Department of Health, (1991). Report on Health and Social Subjects. *Dietary reference values for food, energy and nutrients for the United Kingdom.* Report No. 41, HMSO, UK).

proportion of carbohydrates and refined sugars making up for the decreased fat intake.

With the availability of more data on what young children are eating it is becoming possible to answer some of the questions about how much fat, fibre, and overall energy children in this age group require or can tolerate. However, many questions remain unanswered, and the issue of fat reduction for young children in line with the recommendations for adults, is much debated. Despite this, some policy has evolved and recommendations and dietary guidelines are being made for young children. Of overall importance is meeting their energy needs through the provision of nutrient dense foods. The case for a healthy diet and some of the issues surrounding it are discussed in Chapter 5.

There are certain specific nutritional issues which relate to the preschool years and generally occur in otherwise normal children, but are not manifestations of serious illness; most are self-limiting but nevertheless a serious cause of parental anxiety. These conditions include food fads, toddler diarrhoea, and constipation. Food intake is influenced by family eating patterns, peers, and the media, the latter two become more important as the child gets older. Early food experiences may have an important effect on eating patterns in later life and these appear to be changing as mealtimes are no longer a focal point of family life.

A balanced diet for the toddler

There are several stages in the feeding development of the preschoolchild from messy finger feeding at one year to becoming a competent eater using child-sized cutlery at 4–5 years of age. The intermediate stages include the spoon and bowl used by the 2 year old and the spoon, fork, and plate wielding 3 year old. This is a time when the child will exert his independence and choose what he wants to eat, it is the role of the parent or care giver to provide a healthy diet allowing the child to choose from within this.

What should toddlers be eating? Many people believe that it is important to establish good eating patterns from early childhood as this is likely to establish 'healthy' nutritional patterns for life. Whether there is justification for such a view remains uncertain but on basic principles, the proposition appears sensible. Many British children have extraordinarily unvaried diets and it is possible that this might make them prey to badly balanced food intakes later in life.

Data collected in the recent *National diet and nutrition survey* of children aged 1½ to 4½ years indicates that children are eating the following:

- 51% of energy in the form of carbohydrates mostly as cereal foods with largest amounts provided by white bread, breakfast cereals, and biscuits
- 13% of energy from protein with milk and milk products providing approximately one third of this
- 36% of energy from fat with milk and milk products being a major source followed by cereals, meat products, chips, and other fried potato products
- low intakes of fibre (non starch polysaccharides), average of 6.1 g/day; mainly provided by cereals and smaller amounts from fruits and vegetables

- most frequently consumed vegetables were potato chips, peas, baked beans, and cooked carrots
- most frequently consumed fruits were bananas, apples, and pears with fewer children consuming citrus fruits.

This suggests that the diets of preschoolchildren are generally lower in fibre than is perhaps ideal and do not contain an adequate quantity or variety of fruits and vegetables.

Toddlers are often 'faddy' eaters, with erratic eating habits which makes it difficult to ensure a suitably varied diet. They may eat well at one meal of the day and less well at others. Young children have small appetites and are not generally able to consume all they need without between meal snacks; these are an important part of their nutritional intake. Three meals plus two or three healthy snacks (Table 3.2) should be offered with a variety of foods of differing tastes, textures, and colours which will help maintain the child's interest. Sugary foods should not form a major part of the diet because they make the child reluctant to eat other foods, provide 'empty' calories requiring frequent intake to stave off hunger, and will cause dental caries. To promote a healthy food intake in preschoolchildren the following suggestions can be made:

- provide regular meal times so the child is not too hungry or too tired to eat
- offer a variety of foods of different colours and textures
- offer small portions allowing for second helpings if desired
- keep sweet foods out of sight until savoury foods are eaten but do not use these as a reward
- eat together
- make sure the child is sitting comfortably at the table and has age appropriate utensils
- allow plenty of time to eat
- keep between meal snacks small and give snacks at least 2 hours before meals
- avoid sugar and sweets except as a special treat
- full cream milk should be given to children under the age of 2 years, after that use semi-skimmed; skimmed milk is not recommended under 5 years of age.

Table 3.2. Suitable snack foods for 1–5 year olds

Milk and dairy foods
Whole milk
Cheese cut into cubes, grated or in small slices
Yoghurt, fromage frais

Fruit and vegetables
Fresh fruit e.g. pears, bananas, apple slices, orange segments, kiwi, berries, melon, raisins*
Fresh vegetables e.g. celery sticks*, carrot sticks*, cucumber slices, tomatoes, green or red pepper slices*, broccoli or cauliflower florettes*

Breads and other cereals
Wholemeal bread or toast fingers; plain or with a little butter or margarine
Small sandwiches with fillings such as
　　　　　　　　　　pure fruit spread
　　　　　　　　　　banana
　　　　　　　　　　peanut butter
　　　　　　　　　　lean ham or turkey
　　　　　　　　　　cottage cheese
　　　　　　　　　　cucumber, tomato
wholegrain cereal e.g. Weetabix or Shreddies with whole or semi-skimmed milk

---

*Foods that are hard and do not dissolve can cause choking and should not be given to children under three years of age. Grate or partially cook vegetables for younger children.

A healthy meal plan for toddlers should be based on the *Balance of good health* food guide (see Chapter 5).

The child who 'won't eat'

Many toddlers go through phases of food reluctance or food refusal. These may be due to 'fads' or be part of a strategy of attention seeking. In its less extreme form and when handled sensibly this is part of normal maturation. Transient refusal to eat may be associated with minor illnesses or emotional upsets like the death of a pet. Children on restrictive therapeutic diets may refuse to eat and in some circumstances this can lead to major difficulties.

Food refusal and food fads (toddler strikes) are often part of an overall pattern of behaviour seen in toddlers particularly at around two years of age, a period sometimes called the 'terrible two's'. In most cases the child is well nourished and the problem may be the parent's perception of what they think the child should be eating. Some youngsters have learned to use mealtimes as an excellent way to test out their parents and refuse the food offered precisely because of the anxiety which this provokes. Occasionally the problem is a superficial manifestation of deeper seated family difficulties which should be excluded. The occasional toddler goes on 'hunger-strike' as a response to a new sibling as a form of attention seeking.

Mealtimes can turn into a battle of wills which the child is bound to win. All pleading will be in vain and force-feeding attempts will be utterly counter-productive. By the time the family is referred the situation may have deteriorated to the point where meals have become a nightmare, family relationships have deteriorated, and considerable emotional distress engendered.

The first requirement in these situations is to reassure the parents that the child is not undernourished by accurately measuring and recording height and weight on a centile chart. A detailed dietary history, in the form of a three day food record (Table 3.3), can be very useful in discovering exactly what the child is eating. If the child is thriving and there is no suggestion of any deficiencies, the following suggestions may be helpful:

- offer a balanced variety of food, including known favourites; children have food preferences
- if the meal is refused it should be removed after a reasonable period and no food offered until the next scheduled meal or snack time
- do not force the child to eat
- provide a comfortable, happy mealtime environment
- do not offer sweets as a reward

Table 3.3. Food record chart

Record all food and drink consumed even the smallest amount. Try to be as accurate as possible giving details of the type of food eaten, if a processed food give the manufacturer. Also record the weight or amount in teaspoons, tablespoons, cups, packets, etc. Remember to include all drinks and sweets/snacks.	
Date and time	**Description of food eaten and quantity**
3.4.97 8 a.m. Breakfast 10 a.m. Snack	Rice Crispies—½ small bowl milk (semiskimmed)—4 oz sugar (white)—1 teaspoon 1 small cup apple Juice—4 oz 2 squares Cadbury milk chocolate ½ small banana

- keep snacks small, otherwise the child will not feel hungry at the next mealtime
- offer drinks from a cup only, if the toddler is still having a bottle (an undesirable practice) he will be able to drink more from this. If excessive milk drinking is a problem, limit milk drinks to three cups a day, offer water or dilute juice instead.

As long as the child continues to grow normally, no further action is needed. If growth is sub-optimal the child should be referred to a paediatrician to exclude an organic cause. Even then it is likely that nothing significant will be found. Dietetic advice is useful to ensure that the diet is not defective in some way and to suggest strategies to increase food intake. Sometimes healthy children have unacceptable intakes of energy, vitamins, and minerals. In such cases dietary supplementation is required and a careful growth record should be kept. Quite minor dietary modification may resolve the problem, parents become more relaxed about the food refusal and the child begins to eat normally. Encouraging the child to eat with its peer group at nursery or day care centre is often helpful. In older children (3–4 years of age), simple behaviour modification using star charts and a reward system (positive reinforcement) is worth trying but it is important to include the dietitian, health visitor, or doctor in its implementation. Provided there is no underlying organic disease, the problem always resolves eventually.

Bizarre diets

Toddlers often restrict their intake to a very narrow range of foods, for example diets consisting of milk, crisps, and bread only or baked beans and corn flakes. These bizarre diets will cause great worry to parents and health professionals. In fact such diets often contain much of what the child requires and attempts at forcing the child to eat anything else will not succeed. This pattern often lasts only for a few weeks following which the child eats a different combination of foods. Over a period of time a series of diets not adequate in themselves will provide an over-all balance. A variety of foods should always be offered and patience will eventually be rewarded. Occasionally the problem is due to intake of huge volumes of milk or juice which prevent the child taking other foods. Milk drinks should be restricted to approximately one pint per day allowing room for other foods. Changing the child from a feeder to an ordinary cup can reduce the amount of fluid taken as can offering fluids after meals.

Iron deficiency anaemia

Iron deficiency anaemia (see Chapter 5) is a common problem particularly in the younger preschoolchild. The *National Diet and Nutrition survey* of children aged 1½ to 4 years revealed one in eight of the youngest group of children to be anaemic. The average daily intakes of iron were seen to be well below the RNI.

Health care professionals should be aware of this potential problem and there may be a need to screen for iron-deficiency anaemia in young children, particularly in areas with high prevalence of poverty. Any child who is anaemic should be prescribed iron supplements and dietary advice given regarding foods high in iron (Table 3.4).

Table 3.4. Suggested food sources of iron and vitamin C

Foods high in iron	Foods high in vitamin C
Red meats such as beef, lamb, liver, burgers, sausages, corned beef, other meats including turkey and chicken	Citrus fruits and fruit juices, oranges, satsumers, clementines, mandarin oranges—canned, grapefruit, orange juice, grapefruit juice
Egg yolks	Other fruits including: strawberries, raspberries, kiwi fruit, peaches, nectarines
Cereals and grains: iron fortified breakfast cereals, wholemeal bread	
Beans and pulses such as lentils, baked beans, split peas	Vitamin C fortified juices and squash
Dark green vegetables including spinach, spring cabbage, broccoli	Green vegetables, broccoli, tomatoes
Dried fruits such as apricots, raisins	

Note that drinking tea with iron containing foods will decrease the amount of iron absorbed.

Are supplementary vitamins necessary?

Most infants who are either breast-fed or fed a standard infant formula will at the time of weaning have had an adequate intake of vitamins. The only concerns among normal fullterm babies relate to vitamin C because it is heat labile, and the fat soluble vitamins A and D because they depend to some extent on the level of fat absorption, the presence of stores in the liver and fat depots. Giving a standard vitamin drop preparation containing A, D, and C from about six months of age to all infants as discussed in Chapter 2 seems a reasonable precaution.

Once the child is weaned, the dietary content of these three vitamins will depend on food intake, which may be variable enough to cause problems. Adequate vitamin status should be encouraged through a varied diet and exposure to sunlight; however, if there is any doubt about intake, supplementary vitamins

A, D, and C are recommended until school age (see Table 2.7). It would appear from The *National diet and nutrition survey* that only 5% of preschoolchildren take these vitamin drops, yet many more would benefit from taking them. Children in Britain seem to have very low intakes of fruit and vegetables (major sources of many vitamins) and have intakes of vitamins A and C which are below the RNI. Children in Scotland appear to have lower intakes of these vitamins than children living in England, as do children from lower socio-economic groups probably due to the fact that they consume fewer fruits and vegetables. Those data suggest that the recommendation for vitamin supplements to continue until five years of age is valid.

Most nutritional authorities agree that provided energy and protein intake is adequate and a variety of foods are eaten, deficiency is unlikely. Those parents who feel very strongly about not giving routine supplements can be re-assured that their children will not suffer provided they have good dietary sources of vitamins.

On the other hand there are some parents who seem to become obsessed with the idea that their children are deficient in vitamins. There is no evidence that children on healthy diets or those receiving supplements as recommended are likely to suffer because they have inadequate vitamin intake and there is no case for additional administration.The role of vitamins in the diets of schoolchildren is discussed in Chapter 4.

Nutrients 'at risk'

Children with restricted intakes or unvaried diets may be at risk of nutritional deficiencies. Infants over six months of age and preschoolchildren are particularly at risk of developing iron deficiency anaemia. As discussed in Chapter 5, iron deficiency can be associated with frequent infections, poor weight gain, developmental delay, and behavioural disturbances. It is often associated with late weaning and early introduction of cows' milk and sometimes seen in children who consume large quantities of cows' milk with very few other foods. A varied diet which includes good food sources of iron and adequate vitamin C will prevent this problem. Table 3.4 lists some good sources of iron and vitamin C which are appropriate for the young child.

Toddler diarrhoea

This condition often presents between 6 and 20 months of age and appears to coincide with the period of weaning onto solid foods and usually ceases by the third year of life. The symptoms are increased stool frequency and diarrhoea, with undigested food such as peas and carrots in the stools. These may appear within several hours of ingestion confirming a rapid whole bowel transit time which seems to be a key feature of this disorder. Characteristically the children remain very well, have good appetites, and grow normally.

Causes

There are several possible explanations for toddler diarrhoea. These include recurrent minor infections which the child picks up as a result of increased mobility. The reduction of fat intake associated with weaning is thought to be a factor, because reduced fat speeds up gastric emptying. If this trend is accelerated by placing the child on skimmed or semi-skimmed milk and adding excessive amounts of fibre to the diet, the 'muesli-belt' syndrome of chronic diarrhoea and undernutrition may result. Parents may become fanatical about their own diets and expect children to follow suit. Excessive drinking of fruit juices and squashes in this age group has also been seen to cause toddler diarrhoea. The large amounts of sugar in the juices and particularly high concentrations of fructose cause an osmotic effect in the intestine pulling extra water into the lumen and causing diarrhoea. As well as causing toddler diarrhoea high intakes of juice and squash have also been seen to cause failure to thrive because they replace more nutritious foods and drinks.

Some workers have suggested that toddler diarrhoea may be due to food allergy. In our experience this is unlikely to be the case. Here, as elsewhere, the casual suggestion that a child might have food intolerance, can have serious consequences.

Children with toddler diarrhoea should not be over-investigated. If linear growth and weight gain is satisfactory and the child is otherwise well, apart from stool culture and checking for reducing substances further tests are not indicated.

Management

Management should begin with reassurance of the parents that there is nothing seriously wrong with the child and that the diarrhoea will eventually stop (Fig. 3.1). This in itself will often suffice

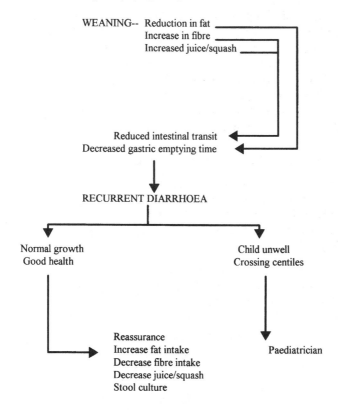

Fig. 3.1. Toddler diarrhoea.

as parents will accept a transient nuisance if they know it is not dangerous. A brief dietary history will establish whether the diet contains excess fibre, inadequate fat, or excess squash or juice and it should be adjusted accordingly.

If there is poor fat intake this may be because the child has given up milk or is drinking skimmed milk. The parents should be advised to increase the intake of whole milk to at least one pint per day. If the child does not like milk, flavourings can be tried to make milkshakes or alternatives such as cheese and yoghurt may be given along with other foods which have a relatively high fat content.

A diet which is too high in fibre will feature many wholegrain cereals, bran supplemented foods, and sometimes added bran. Pure bran should not be given to young children and may need to be reduced in any child with diarrhoea.

If toddler diarrhoea appears to be associated with the child drinking large amounts of squash or fruit juice, intake of these should be reduced. Water or very dilute squash or juice are acceptable drinks for young children as long as they do not replace other necessary foods including an appropriate intake of milk.

Dietary intervention for toddler diarrhoea will therefore include:

* encouraging a healthy well balanced diet
* increasing intake of whole milk to approximately one pint daily
* decreasing intake of high-fibre foods, avoiding added bran
* limiting drinks of juice or squash and making sure it is well diluted with water.

Drug therapy to slow bowel movements has been advocated but it is our view that this is best avoided, unless diarrhoea is causing severe social disruption such an exclusion from nursery school.

Constipation

From about two years of age faecal retention often associated with soiling becomes increasingly common. In some children the cause is excessive milk drinking, often still from the bottle, with a poor food intake. Important principles of treatment include:

• evacuate the bowel at regular intervals following meals
• increasing faecal bulk through diet
• use of laxatives (such as lactulose)
• behaviour modification using star charts and positive reinforcement
• increased fluid intake
• increased exercise

Laxatives should not be seen as a long-term solution but as a stepping stone to the establishment of a normal bowel habit.

It would be a mistake to place too much reliance on diet alone in severe cases. No doubt, a general increase in fibre and fluid intake will reduce the prevalence of constipation, but those who have attempted to treat large numbers of severely constipated and soiling younger children will know that its role is at best supportive. On the other hand simple less severe constipation will respond quite well to a high-fibre diet. This requires changes in the eating habits of the whole family towards a greater fibre intake and more healthy food choices. It is counter-productive for all the family members to tuck into slices of white bread while the child is left miserably contemplating a thick, and to him unappetizing, lump of rough brown loaf. If the brown bread is so good, why isn't everybody eating it?!

The star chart approach used for general management of constipation may also be useful in achieving some increased fibre intake in younger children. Stars are awarded each time the child eats a portion containing fibre.

This dietary programme is combined with behaviour modification directed towards achieving a regular bowel habit. The child is encouraged to sit on the toilet every day after meals, to make use of the peristaltic reaction (gastro-colic reflex) which occurs after eating, and a star awarded for this. Additionally, stars are gained by successful defaecation and absence of soiling. A contract is agreed whereby once the child has achieved an appropriate number of stars a reward will be given by one of the parents.

Many of the families with children with truly resistant constipation and soiling have major social and emotional problems. For them a radical dietary change only adds to their general burdens. These children tend to remain constipated for years and it is not clear what eventually happens to them. Input from the child mental health team may be helpful.

The high-fibre diet

Dietary fibre consists of non-starch polysaccharides which are complexes of cellulose. They are mainly derived from the cell walls of plants and generally passed through the intestine in an undigested form and are therefore not absorbed. The aim of a high-fibre diet is to include increased amounts of unrefined and fibrous foods along with a good fluid intake, whilst maintaining adequate levels of all nutrients. As we have already discussed, high-fibre diets can be problematic in this age group and care should be taken to avoid nutrient deficiencies. All preschoolchildren requiring a high-fibre diet should be referred to a dietitian to make sure that the diet is nutritionally adequate. The RNIs do not make a specific recommendation as to the amount of fibre young children should be eating. In the United States recommendations have been made for appropriate fibre intakes for children, and a simple formula developed as follows:

'American children over two years of age should consume a minimum amount of dietary fibre equivalent to age (in grams) plus 5 g/day'.

Therefore a 2 year old should consume 7 g/day and a 4 year old 9 g/day. Some general recommendations for increasing fibre in the diet include:

- replace white bread with wholemeal, granary, or high bran varieties; high-fibre white bread is also an acceptable alternative
- start the day with a cereal high in fibre (see Table 3.5); or mix a high-fibre cereal with other cereals (for young children avoid those containing whole nuts)
- eat more vegetables, try raw vegetables and leave skins on when acceptable

Table 3.5. Fibre content of selected foods

Food	Serving size	Approx. fibre content (g)
Cereals		
All-Bran	30 g	7.2
Bran Flakes	30 g	3.9
Weetabix	30 g	2.9
Shreddies	30 g	2.8
muesli	30 g	1.9
Rice Krispies	30 g	0.2
Breads		
wholemeal	30 g (1 slice)	1.7
granary	30 g (1 slice)	1.3
white	30 g (1 slice)	0.5
Vegetables		
peas	50 g	2.6
carrots	50 g	1.2
green beans	50 g	0.9
Fruit		
apple (with skin)	1	2.1
banana	1 small	1.3
pear (with skin)	1	2.4
Pasta (cooked)		
wholemeal	45 g	1.6
white	45 g	0.5
Rice (cooked)		
brown	100 g	0.8
white	100 g	0.1

- eat plenty of fruit, including the skins; dried fruits are particularly high in fibre
- try wholemeal pasta and brown rice instead of the white varieties

• use wholemeal flour in baking and purchase products containing wholemeal flour
• drink plenty of fluid especially water or very dilute fruit juice; at least 6–8 cups a day is recommended.

These recommendations for increasing fibre should be incorporated into a general well-balanced diet based on the needs of the individual child. Table 3.6 provides a sample high fibre menu for a young child. It is important to remember that high-fibre foods are filling and other nutrient dense foods need to be included in the diet. It is often only necessary to make one or two changes to the child's diet, for example including a high-fibre cereal and changing to wholemeal bread or increasing fruit and vegetable intake to four or five servings daily. As fibre soaks up water it is essential that fluid intake is increased at the same time as increasing fibre intake.

Dental caries

Dental caries appears to be decreasing in children, probably related to generally better oral hygiene; however, in some small subgroups of the preschool population it has increased. For dental caries to develop carbohydrate, bacteria, and a susceptible tooth must be present. The bacteria acts on the carbohydrate to produce acids which in turn demineralize the tooth enamel. Several reports have shown an increase in dental caries in children who are bottle fed for prolonged periods, often after the age of two years. These children are given many bottles of milk or juice each day and allowed to suck on them constantly. This provides a perfect situation for the bacteria in the plaque and leads to tooth decay (Fig. 3.2). Increased dental caries has also been seen in children who require long-term liquid medications, if these contain sugars.

Dietary treatment should include removal of concentrated sugars from the diet, changing from a bottle to a cup, using sugar-free medications and promotion of good eating habits. When sugary foods are eaten they should be eaten at a mealtime with other foods, not as snacks. Good oral hygiene is very important

Table 3.6. Sample menu for a 2 year old

	Fibre approx. (g)	Kcal approx.
Breakfast		
30 g Rice Krispies	0.2	110
100 ml whole milk	0	70
orange juice—50 cc		
diluted with water	0	18
Morning snack		
½ slice wholemeal bread	0.9	32
1 teaspoon butter or margarine	0	45
100 ml whole milk	0	70
Lunch		
1 slice wholemeal bread	1.7	64
1 slice ham	0	36
15 g cheese	0	60
1 teaspoon butter or margarine	0	45
apple juice—diluted with water	0	18
yoghurt—low fat, smooth	tr.	135
Afternoon snack		
1 banana	1.3	55
100 ml whole milk	0	70
Dinner		
Shepherds pie		145
2 oz mince	0	
2 oz mashed potato	0.5	
carrots—25 g	0.6	6
1 digestive biscuit	0.3	70
½ pear	1.2	
100 ml milk	0	70
Total	6.7	1119
Recommended	7	1165
	(U.S. recommendation	(EAR)
	5 g + 1 g/year)	

along with regular dental check-ups and treatment as necessary. Some suggestions to prevent toddler caries include:

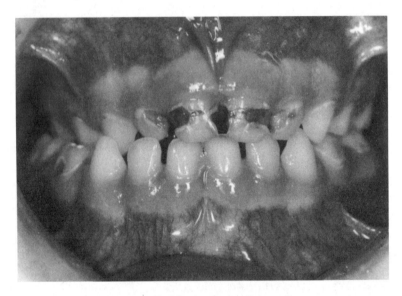

Fig. 3.2. Toddler bottle feeding caries.

- avoid bottle-feeding after one year of age
- do not use bottles as comforters or as juice feeders
- do not put a child to bed with a bottle
- avoid bottle-propping
- do not allow a breast-fed infant to 'comfort suckle' throughout the night
- graduate to a cup as soon as the child is able to use one.

Further reading

HMSO (1995). *National diet and nutrition survey.* Children aged 1½ to 4½ years. Volume 1: Report of the diet and nutrition survey. HMSO, London.

Lifshitz, F. and Tarim, O. (1996). Considerations about dietary fat restrictions for children. *Journal of Nutrition*, 1031S–41S.

Smith, M.M. and Lifshitz, F. (1994). Excess fruit juice consumption as a contributing factor in nonorganic failure to thrive. *Pediatrics*, **93**, (3), 438–43.

Williams, C.L., Bollella, M. and Wynder, E.L. (1995). A new recommendation for dietary fiber in childhood. *Pediatrics*, **96**, (5), 985–8.

4

....

The schoolchild and adolescent

Schoolchildren and adolescents in Britain are taller and heavier than in the past and the secular trend for increasing body size continues. This has been interpreted as evidence that the population is healthier than ever before and that nutritional standards continue to improve. However, there is growing concern that changes in social policy and in life-style may put at least some schoolchildren and adolescents at risk because they could have subclinical nutritional deficiencies. In addition there is the possibility that the increased intake of energy and fat, particularly animal fat may be predisposing the younger generation to an increased risk of cardio-vascular disease.

A balanced diet for the schoolchild

The years from five until adolescence mark a period of slow but steady growth with a corresponding increase in nutritional requirements as outlined in the reference nutrient intakes (RNIs). These are divided into age-related groupings reflecting growth rate. Table 4.1 summarizes some of the RNIs for children and adolescents. It is important to remember that these are

Table 4.1. Reference nutrient intakes of selected nutrients for schoolchildren and adolescent

Nutrient (per day)	7–10 years		Boys 11–14 years	Girls 11–14 years	Boys 15–18 years	Girls 15–18 years
	M	F				
Energy (EAR) (kcal)	1970	1740	2220	1845	2755	2110
Protein (g)	28.3		42.1	41.2	55.2	45.0
Thiamin (mg)	0.7		0.9	0.7	1.1	0.8
Riboflavin (mg)	1.0		1.2	1.1	1.3	1.1
Folate (µg)	150		200	200	200	200
Vitamin C (mg)	30		35	35	40	40
Vitamin A (µg)	500		600	600	700	600
Calcium (mmol) (mg)	13.8 (550)		25.0 (1000)	20.0 (800)	25.0 (1000)	20.0 (800)
Iron (µmol) (mg)	160 (8.7)		200 (11.3)	260 (14.8)	200 (11.3)	260 (14.8)

EAR: estimated average requirement.

(Adapted from: Department of Health (1991). Report on Health and Social Subjects. *Dietary reference values for food, energy and nutrients for the United Kingdom*. Report No. 41, HMSO, UK).

guidelines and not specific requirements for each individual. Children may have lower or higher needs of certain nutrients particularly during differing periods of growth; however, the RNIs encompass the needs of most healthy children. RNIs for fat, carbohydrate, and fibre intakes are not available, but some guidelines have been made as discussed in Chapter 5 (pp. 95–100). A formula for a suitable fibre intake has been adopted in the United States and is described in Chapter 3 (pp. 65 and 66).

A 1983 survey of the diets of British schoolchildren revealed that although children consumed adequate intakes of many nutrients a large number did not achieve RNIs for iron and calcium. Other important nutritional aspects of the diets of schoolchildren highlighted in this study included:

• schoolchildren generally ate many foods that were high in fat and sugar
• the main sources of dietary energy were bread, chips, milk, biscuits, meat products, cakes, and puddings
• approximately 37%–38% energy was from fat and over ¾ of the children had intakes greater than the recommended 35%
• children ate lower than desirable intakes of fruits and vegetables
• differences were seen in food choices and nutrient intakes between girls and boys; girls ate more fruit and fruit juices whereas boys ate more chips, milk, breakfast cereals, and baked beans. Older girls had lower intakes of calcium and riboflavin (below RNI), mainly because of reduced milk intake.

Subsequent smaller studies have supported this information, and it would appear that the diets of British schoolchildren are too high in fat, saturated fat, and sugar and too low in iron, calcium, and dietary fibre and probably low in antioxidant nutrients.

Many changes occur in a child's life when formal education begins. The noon meal is frequently taken at school and the environment in which food is eaten will be very different from home. Getting to school on time can interfere with breakfast, children may be unwilling to get up in time to eat and some busy parents may not have time to provide their children with an adequate breakfast. As children become more independent they are increasingly responsible for making their own food choices and parental influence decreases. Children of working parents may be left on their own after school to select their evening meal and there seems to be a trend away from the family meal where everyone sits down to eat together.

Schoolchildren should consume a diet based on a wide variety of foods as outlined in the *Balance of good health* (Fig. 5.1) and the eight guidelines for a healthy diet (Table 5.1). A healthy diet should include a variety of:

• starchy foods such as wholemeal bread, potatoes, pasta, and rice; at least one of these foods at each meal
• vegetables and fruit, eating skin whenever possible; a minimum of five servings a day is a good guideline for all age groups
• meat or alternatives including beans and legumes, fish, poultry, eggs; one serving twice a day
• semi-skimmed milk, low fat yoghurt, fromage frais, cheese; aim for 1 pint of milk daily (200 ml (1/3 pint) = 1 yoghurt = 30 g (1 oz) cheese)
• sugar and fats, these are 'sometimes foods', use in small amounts occasionally.

Nutritional issues in schoolchildren

Schoolchildren have changing nutritional needs which vary according to the level of growth and various nutritional problems can arise. These include undernutrition which is characterized by poor growth and in anaemia, particularly in children from low income families or where a poor diet is eaten. Rickets is seen in Asian children and in children who are on unusual diets. Other problems include obesity (see Chapter 10) and dental caries.

Anaemia

Anaemia can occur in schoolchildren when dietary iron intake is poor and is more often seen in low income families or in situations where the child has eating habits which differ from the normal e.g. vegetarian. Iron deficiency anaemia is discussed in Chapter 5 (pp 102–4). It is important that children who have iron deficiency anaemia are encouraged to eat foods rich in iron (Table 3.4). Unfortunately, these are often unpopular with children and many refuse to eat red meats, green vegetables, or fresh fruits. Alternative foods or methods of serving high iron foods can be found and unpopular foods can sometimes be presented in a more acceptable way or disguised in other foods. Some suggestions include:

- puréed red meats or lentils can be added to gravy or soup
- iron fortified cereal can be mixed into yoghurt or puréed fruits
- dried fruits can be added to baked goods such as cakes or biscuits
- dark green vegetables can be puréed and added to stews, soups, or gravies.

Poor meal habits

With increasing age children are more likely to skip meals especially breakfast. This will reduce nutrient intakes which are difficult to make up later in the day and may result in nutrient deficiencies. Several studies have indicated that breakfast plays an important role in the intellectual and physical performance of schoolchildren. Children who do not eat breakfast have been shown to have changes in brain function, particularly in the speed of information retrieval in working memory and this is especially true in children who are already undernourished.

Children should be encouraged to eat a nutritionally balanced breakfast every morning and some suggestions for suitable choices include:

- high-fibre cereal such as Weetabix, Bran Flakes, Shreddies or Mini Shredded Wheat with fruit (banana, strawberries, dried fruit) and semi-skimmed milk
- porridge made with semi-skimmed milk, a glass of fresh orange or grapefruit juice
- wholemeal toast spread thinly with butter or marg egg or a slice of cheese, and some fresh fruit or f

- wholemeal or granary bread, toasted, with butter or margarine and a little jam or fruit spread, and a glass of semi-skimmed milk
- fruit yoghurt, wholemeal toast with butter or margarine, glass of fresh orange juice.

Dental caries

Although the prevalence of dental caries has declined in recent years, 50% of children still experience tooth decay before their permanent teeth appear. The decline in decay is related to the fluoridation of water supplies and toothpaste, with the major cause of caries being the consumption of sugary foods especially as between meal snacks. Foods most likely to promote dental caries include:

- sweets
- toffee and other sticky foods such as dates or raisins
- chocolates
- acid foods e.g. citrus fruits and drinks, cola drinks.

Eating these foods at a mealtime lessens their cariogenicity, as does eating alkaline foods such as cheese, milk, or peanuts at the end of a meal. Frequent snacks increase the risk of caries and constant snacking should be avoided.

Fluoride supplements are recommended in areas where water is not fluoridated (Table 4.2).

Table 4.2. Flouride supplements

Age	Water content < 300 μg/l (0.3 ppm)	Water content 300–700 μg/l (0.3–0.7 ppm)
0–6 months	0	0
6 months–2 years	250 μg/day	0
2–4 years	500 μg/day	250 μg/day
> 4 years	1 mg/day	500 μg/day

Note: doses are given for flouride ion.

School meals

In the UK, the 1980 Education Act made major changes to the laws governing the provision of school meals. Local authorities are no longer required to provide meals of a certain nutritional standard at a fixed price. Prior to 1980 the school meal was required to provide a third of a child's nutritional intake. More recently in 1988 the Local Government Act required all school meals to undergo a competitive tender process which has resulted in considerable variations in the standards of school meals. There is strong opinion that the government should adopt new guidelines for the nutritional content of school meals, not only to improve the nutritional status of undernourished children but also to support the nutrition education component of the National Curriculum, thereby providing a complete approach to nutrition. An adequate school lunch, by preventing children from being hungry may also influence intellectual performance.

The consequences of the changes in the school meal system have been:

• there is no guarantee that meals provided meet a required nutritional standard, and therefore that the child will receive an adequate meal
• although there may be a wide choice designed to attract custom this may not educate children into healthy eating habits if the food choices are high in fat and sugar and low in fibre and vitamins
• children are free to spend dinner money elsewhere.

On the positive side, many schools are working hard to offer healthy meals. Nutritional guidelines have been set out by many local authorities with input from dietitians and school meals which are attractive to children and meet healthy eating policies are being provided. School meal departments should be encouraged to link with teachers to complement and reinforce nutrition education.

Problems with school meals include inadequate time available, particularly for young children who are slow eaters. If a child has to queue for a long time to obtain his meal there may be little time left to eat it and the choice of food may be limited. In many schools there is a lack of suitable meals for minority groups including vegetarians. In older schoolchildren the temptation to skip school lunch and eat out at a fast food take-away can mean that an unbalanced meal is eaten. Parents may be unaware of what their children are eating and so are not able to make up deficiencies at home. Particularly at risk are children from less privileged homes. All these problems are compounded by the growing tendency for convenience foods to be eaten and for increasing consumption of high fat snack foods, often obtained from school vending machines. The British Dietetic Association in its position statement on school meals has made the following recommendations:

- government supported nutrition guidelines should be introduced
- vending machines in schools should provide healthy food choices
- State Registered Dietitians should be involved in the development of nutritional guidelines and in the implementation of the nutrition aspects of the National Curriculum.

Children require more nutrition education and assistance in choosing a healthy meal. Table 4.3 provides guidelines for selecting a healthy school lunch. Many children take packed lunches to school and to add healthy variety try:

- wholemeal or granary bread, rolls, pitta bread, high-fibre white bread, crackers
- fillings such as egg mayonnaise and cress, tuna fish and cucumber, cottage cheese and pineapple, cheese and tomato or beetroot, chicken and salad or ham and coleslaw
- sticks of raw vegetables, yoghurt, fromage frais, fresh or dried fruit
- drinks of water, fresh fruit juice, semi-skimmed milk, or low sugar squash.

The provision of subsidized school milk has recently been reduced; however, it is still available to nursery and primary schoolchildren and can be utilized as part of the school lunch or at another time in the school day.

Table 4.3. Guidelines for choosing a healthy school lunch

Always have a protein food. This may be meat, fish, eggs, cheese, beans or lentils.	Try not to have pies, burgers, or sausages every day as these are high in fat.
Choose at least one starchy food at each meal which will help fill you up, such as bread rolls, jacket potatoes, boiled potatoes, pasta, or rice.	Chips can be eaten occasionally, but are too high in fat to eat daily.
Add at least one portion of vegetable to each meal. This may be raw or cooked vegetable or salad.	
Have a piece of fruit after a main meal—either fresh, dried, or tinned in fruit juice.	

Adapted with permission from *Food for the school years*, (Paediatric Group, British Dietetic Association 1993).

Diet and behaviour

Food intolerance and dietary additives may rarely be responsible for behaviour problems including hyperkinetic disorders (hyperactivity or attention deficit disorder) in some children and this is discussed in Chapter 9. Other dietary factors which are thought to have effects on behaviour and intelligence in schoolchildren are sucrose and supposed vitamin deficiency.

Sucrose

Despite health education to promote a reduction in sugar intake, studies of British children's eating habits show no decrease. Sugar is considered to provide 'empty calories', increase dental caries, and is not a necessary food item. A reduction in sugar intake as outlined in healthy eating recommendations, is desirable for the whole population.

Dietary sugar and behaviour problems
Some writers have claimed that an increased intake of sucrose and the sweetener aspartame may cause learning and behaviour

difficulties in school children. A double blind controlled trial with two groups of children (25 normal preschoolchildren, and 23 school age children said by parents to be sensitive to sugar) failed to show any effect of sucrose or aspartame on children's behaviour or cognitive function, even with intakes in excess of typical dietary levels.

It has also been claimed that sucrose may cause hyperkinesis or aggravate symptoms in already hyperactive children. However, current research indicates that there is little or no valid evidence to support the views that a high sucrose intake is an important cause of behaviour disturbance, either by causing hypoglycaemia or through some other mechanism.

Vitamins and minerals

Most children consume adequate amounts of vitamins and minerals in their diets and vitamin supplements are not considered necessary. Surveys of the diets of schoolchildren, as discussed previously, have revealed deficits in some nutrients and in those children at risk for deficiencies supplements are appropriate.

There have been studies suggesting that supplementing children's diets with megadoses of vitamins and minerals may improve non-verbal intelligence. These findings have not been substantiated and more evidence is needed to prove them valid. In fact there is a serious danger that supplementing may lead to vitamin toxicity especially for the fat-soluble vitamins which are not excreted from the body. Excess intake of vitamin A can cause hypertension and brain injury while vitamin D poisoning will lead to hypercalcaemia and renal damage. Water-soluble vitamins are safer than fat-soluble ones as any excess intake is excreted in the urine; however, huge doses of ascorbic acid can cause haematuria and a massive intake of pyridoxine (B_6) has been associated with peripheral neuropathy.

The antioxidant vitamins C, E, and carotene may play an important role in long-term development of disease as discussed in Chapter 5.

There are considerable attractions both for parents and health professionals in trying to ascribe often intractable and worrying problems to causes which might be amenable to relatively simple solutions. Parents with children who are not achieving what might be expected of them, or those whose behaviour has become intolerable are likely to grasp at the straws provided by potential 'cures' which are simple, cheap, and apparently harmless. It is not easy for parents to accept that underachievement or disturbed behaviour might be inherited or environmental.

Establishing a scientifically valid link between dietary deficiencies (or excess) and conditions which are usually multifactorial in their origins is a notoriously tricky area for investigation.

Preparations of vitamins can be freely bought from health food shops and pharmacies. Provided parents do not overdose their children with vitamins A or D it is unlikely that this form of supplementation will do much harm. Currently, there seems to be no justification for providing multiple vitamin/mineral supplementation to children over five years of age at public expense.

The adolescent

Because of the rapid growth spurt during adolescence energy and nutrient requirements are greatly increased. The peak period of growth is between 11 and 15 years of age for girls and between 13 and 16 years for boys. Girls accumulate relatively more fat and boys more lean body mass. Overall boys increase their total body mass much more dramatically than girls and so RNI values deviate increasingly from about 11 years of age. The amount of energy required will depend on the degree of physical activity in which the individual is engaged and this varies considerably. Many adolescents have low dietary intakes of calcium and iron and other possible 'at risk nutrients' include zinc and folate.

Adolescent eating patterns

Adolescents are eating more away from the home environment and there is an increasing tendency towards snack foods, some of which are high in fat. Those who do not eat school lunch and eat out of the school environment have been seen to have diets of poor nutritional quality. Adolescence is a time in which a transition occurs from child to adult eating behaviour and experimentation with new eating habits is common. Some adolescents may opt for vegetarianism out of serious principle and should be given every assistance in establishing their new way of life on a sound nutritional footing.

Food faddism based on misconceptions about food may lead to poor food choice and suboptimal nutrition. Fortunately most fads are short term and have no lasting ill effects. Nutrition education is important because of its role in preventing adult disease and because it provides a sound basis for future parenthood. However, due to the nature of adolescence this is difficult as suggestions made by an adult are likely to be viewed with suspicion and ignored, at least at first.

'Nutrients at risk'

The two main nutrients at risk during adolescence are iron and calcium and low intakes of these nutrients are common. Iron requirements increase in adolescence particularly in girls with the onset of menstruation. Foods high in iron and vitamin C are not usually found in preferred snack foods and convenience meals and therefore the intake of these nutrients is likely to be low. Adolescents who consume milk and dairy products are unlikely to have a calcium deficiency, but those who do not may fail to meet their increased needs for this nutrient.

Other nutrients which may be low in the diets of adolescents include zinc (a nutrient found in many of the foods containing iron) and folate which is found in dark green vegetables and citrus fruits.

Adolescents should be encouraged to eat a well-balanced diet based on the *Balance of good health* and health promotion in schools should include nutrition education.

Nutritional issues in adolescence

There are several nutritional issues during adolescence including eating disorders, obesity (see Chapter 10), teenage pregnancy, and as sports are promoted as part of a healthy life-style, nutrition issues relating to extensive training may become important. Studies have shown that many adolescents follow slimming regimens and some of these may be very restrictive and nutritionally deficient. At a time of rapid growth these regimens can cause growth impairment and delay of pubertal development. Dieting is more common in girls but is also seen in boys. Appropriate advice on sensible weight reduction should be given, with an emphasis on practical dietary changes to fit in with the adolescent life-style.

Anorexia nervosa

This term describes a state in which aversion to food is global and so severe as to cause dangerous weight loss, associated with amenorrhoea in girls in whom the condition is more common. Some cases of prepubertal anorexia nervosa occur and anorexia is sometimes seen in older women.

If there is a threat to life because of malnutrition, admission to hospital is necessary. The management will include psychiatric treatment in conjunction with dietary manipulation to achieve a safe weight through adequate nutrition. The regimen may include nasogastric feeding, dietary supplements, and a graded reintroduction of food.

Bulimia nervosa

Bulimia nervosa involves a cycle of binge eating followed by vomiting and laxative use whilst usually maintaining body weight. The binge and purge cycle often occupies the sufferer for many hours of the day. They are obsessed with food and have a distorted body image. Figure 4.1 illustrates this cycle. Treatment for bulimia is usually effective and involves a multi-disciplinary team approach usually with some aspect of behaviour therapy and nutritional education to promote a regular eating pattern.

Teenage pregnancy

Teenage pregnancy is increasing in Britain. Pregnancy makes considerable additional demands on the body at a time when the

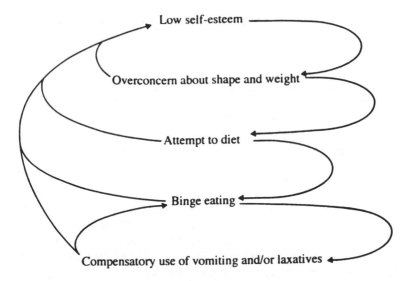

Fig. 4.1. Maintenance of the bullimic condition.

nutritional demands for adolescent growth are at their greatest. Nutrition plays a very important role in the outcome of the pregnancy and practical, cost conscious nutritional advice along with information on food preparation is essential.

Physical activity

Teenagers involved in physical training schedules often adopt bizarre eating patterns based on unsound nutritional information. Diets may include very high protein intakes or excessive doses of vitamins and minerals. Eating times can be disrupted by training schedules and expensive liquid diets may be consumed in preference to a meal. Inadequate nutrition can be a problem. Sensible healthy eating advice is important for these adolescents and if presented in an appropriate manner is well accepted as part of improving athletic performance.

On the other hand many adolescents do not exercise and there is a need to promote more physical activity as part of overall health promotion for the general population.

Further reading

British Dietetic Association (1993). *School meals: a position paper.* British Dietetic Association, Birmingham.

Paediatric Group, British Dietetic Association (1993). *Food for the school years.* British Dietetic Association, Birmingham.

Pollitt, E. (1995). Does breakfast make a difference in school? *Journal of the American Dietetic Association*, **95**, 1134–39.

Wolraich, M.L., Lindgren, S.D., Stumbo, P.J. Stegink, L.D., Applebaum, M.I., and Kiritsg, M.C. (1994). Effects of diets high in sucrose or aspartame on the behaviour and cognitive performance of children. *New England Journal of Medicine*, **330**, 301–7.

5

....

Healthy eating to prevent adult disease

Many people believe that 'healthy eating' can help promote good health, and undoubtedly dietary factors play a role in many different diseases. Whereas the mechanisms of illness in deficiency states (e.g. iron, vitamins, trace elements) are relatively well understood, other diseases such as cancer appear to have a more complex relationship to diet. There is considerable scope for debate and discussion regarding what constitutes a healthy diet, and no absolute agreement. Perhaps it is not surprising that the public perception is of constantly changing 'food for health' messages, and of interminable disagreements among the 'experts'. This is no more than a reflection of our limited, albeit developing insights into disease and nutrition, coupled with the fact that it is often genuinely difficult to translate new scientific findings into public health policy and dietary recommendations. However, the COMA reports from the Department of Health and other recent summaries of the scientific literature represent progress in this area.

On an international scale, The World Health Organisation has participated in a series of conferences which have examined world-wide dietary traditions that historically have been associated with good health, for example the 'Mediterranean diet' which reflects food patterns of Crete, other parts of Greece, and southern Italy in the early 1960s. In these areas, adult life expectancy was amongst the highest in the world, and rates of coronary heart disease, certain cancers, and some other diet-related diseases were among the lowest in the world.

The health of the nation

In 1993 the UK government adopted a White paper entitled '*The health of the nation*'. The stated objective of the proposals within the White Paper was to 'add years to life and life to years'. Five 'key areas' were identified for immediate action:

• coronary heart disease and stroke
• cancers
• mental health
• HIV/AIDS and sexual health
• accidents.

As good nutrition was seen to be an important contributor to positive health, a Nutrition Task Force was set up by the Department of Health in order to advise ministers on action required to achieve the *Health of the Nation* dietary targets. The eight guidelines for a healthy diet (Table 5.1) were developed,

Table 5.1. The eight guidelines for a healthy diet

---
1. Enjoy your food.
2. Eat a variety of different foods.
3. Eat the right amount to be a healthy weight.
4. Eat plenty of foods rich in starch and fibre.
5. Don't eat too much fat.
6. Don't eat sugary foods too often.
7. Look after the vitamins and minerals in your food.
8. If you drink alcohol, keep within sensible limits—this guideline does not apply to children, but some teenagers drink alcohol and should keep to sensible levels which are lower than for adults.

Fruit and vegetables   Bread, other cereals and potatoes

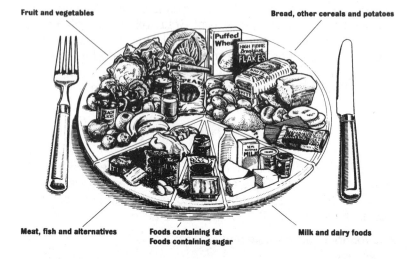

Meat, fish and alternatives   Foods containing fat   Milk and dairy foods
                                Foods containing sugar

Health Education Authority, reproduced with permission

NB. Exact number of servings and amounts will vary according to age and energy needs. Consult a State Registered Dietitian. The proportions from the fruit and vegetable and the bread, other cereals and potatoes groups should make up the largest component of the diet. Further information available from HEA, see further reading section.

Fig. 5.1. The balance of good health.

followed by a pictorial food guide in the form of a tilted plate (Fig. 5.1) to help consumers in selecting a balanced diet. Explicit dietary guidelines were elaborated in an earlier Department of Health publication, *Dietary reference values for food energy and nutrients for the United Kingdom* published in 1991. These included:

- a reduction in the total fat content of the diet, particularly by reducing the amount of saturated fat; and
- changes in the pattern of carbohydrate consumption, with a decrease in simple sugars and an increase in complex carbohydrates (starch and non-starch polysaccharides).

Implications for children

Although the consequences of an unhealthy diet may not be apparent for many years, it seems sensible to encourage healthy eating from early childhood. However, children are not small adults and proposals which may be very reasonable for adults may have harmful effects on the young. For example many health workers will be familiar with the toddler from the 'muesli-belt' who is failing to thrive and has diarrhoea as a result of being on a 'healthy' low fat/high-fibre diet. Well motivated actions may have untoward consequences and a sense of perspective is required.

Much epidemiological evidence has been presented to suggest that many conditions in adulthood relate primarily to poor growth during fetal development and early infancy. A novel and challenging model of the origins of adult disease in which nutritional influences play a crucial role is offered in the 'Barker hypothesis' (discussed later). One of the implications of this hypothesis is that disease prevention strategies might be much more effective if focused on nutrition in early life rather than persuading adults to make life-style changes. This, however, remains a controversial issue at the present time.

Cardio-vascular disease

Diet is not the only, or necessarily the most important factor in the causation of cardio-vascular disease. Nor may events in early childhood be a very large factor when compared with the unhealthy life-style which can be acquired during later childhood and adolescence. The influence which parents have on their children in other ways may be more important than persuading them to drink skimmed milk. For example smoking in the presence of children whilst simultaneously trying to persuade them to consume huge volumes of high-fibre foods, would not be a rational way of preventing a coronary in later life!

The origins of atherosclerosis

Atherosclerosis is a degenerative disease of the walls of arteries, particularly the aorta, the coronary arteries, and the cerebral vessels. Cholesterol-rich fatty deposits are characteristic, forming a material called plaque. The complete obstruction of coronary or cerebral vessels which is the end stage of the process is often due to thrombosis occurring at the site of plaque. Consequently, there are two distinct phases to the disease, a long process of plaque formation which may take place over many years, followed by acute occlusion of the vessel due to thrombosis. There is little doubt that in certain individuals who are particularly at risk, atherosclerosis may begin at a very young age. Individuals who are homozygous for familial hypercholesterolaemia, for example, may die of coronary occlusion during adolescence. Heavily smoking teenagers have been shown to develop severe atherosclerosis by early adulthood. Autopsies carried out on very young men killed during the Korean War showed quite advanced atheroma. The question is whether diet is the primary factor in this early disease and how soon an 'atherogenic diet' will produce potentially dangerous lesions.

Fatty streaks are found in the aortas of young children (3 years of age), but not in their coronary arteries. They occur equally commonly in children from populations who do not have a significant incidence of adult atherosclerosis and appear to be the site of future disease rather than evidence that it is already present. Fatty streaks are apparently reversible. Coronary artery fatty streaks have been found in pre-adolescents (after 10 years of age) from populations with a high incidence of atherosclerosis and some authorities regard them as more indicative of true vascular disease, and evidence that risk factors for atheroma are present.

The crucial event in the pathogenesis of atherosclerosis seems to be the conversion of fatty streaks to atheromatous plaque which begins in later childhood (after 10 years) and during adolescence in 'at risk' groups. There are no convincing data to suggest that irreversible change occurs before then. There is evidence that eliminating risk factors in individuals with quite advanced atherosclerosis will halt the progression of the disease and reduce the risk of catastrophic events such as stroke or coronary infarction. For example people who have had a coronary episode can improve their outlook if they change their lifestyle, by exercising more, changing their diets, and stopping smoking. It is not self-evident that dramatic changes in the eating habits of very young children is imperative, and it is very important not to lose sight of other preventable factors. Teenage smoking may be a far more serious cause of future vascular disease.

Risk factors for atherosclerosis

How much it is reasonable to modify childrens' diets depends on specific dietary risk factors for vascular disease and to what extent they operate from childhood. The possible interrelationships of risk factors is illustrated in Fig. 5.2. It will be noted that diet plays only a part in the overall picture, but a very important

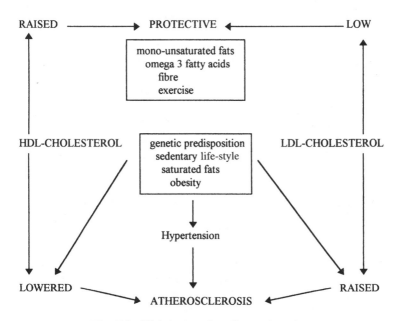

Fig. 5.2. Risk factors for atherosclerosis.

part because its consequences are potentially preventable. Some of the main pieces in the 'jigsaw' are discussed below.

Serum lipids

As a 'hunter-gatherer', man's 'natural diet' was essentially omnivorous including seeds, roots, berries, and fruits supplemented with occasional meat. Animals in the wild are generally lean so dietary fat would be relatively high in unsaturated fatty acids and low in saturated fatty acids. The western diet has moved towards a much greater intake of animal fats, partly because we eat more meat, and partly because meat from animals reared commercially and selected for rapid weight gain contains more structural fat. A diet high in saturated fats correlates both with cholesterol levels and with coronary heart disease levels found in a community.

Cholesterol is essential in the metabolism of steroid hormones, bile salts, and cell membranes, and triglyceride plays a major part in energy storage in the body. Cholesterol is carried in the plasma in various forms depending on the nature of the neutral fats to which it is attached. Fat and cholesterol are transported through the circulation by carriers called lipoproteins:

- atherogenic low density lipoprotein (LDL)—70% of circulating cholesterol
- cardioprotective high density lipoprotein (HDL)
- high levels of triglycerides (TGs) with low levels of HDL increase risk of heart disease.

Total cholesterol is associated with atherosclerosis because high blood cholesterol levels are usually due to increases in LDL.

Both LDL and HDL fractions can be influenced by dietary intake, although dietary cholesterol has only a small effect on LDL cholesterol in the blood. High levels of unsaturated fats in the diet such as sunflower and certain other vegetable oils tend to raise HDL and lower LDL-cholesterol levels. People from Mediterranean countries with high intakes of olive oil have low LDL and high HDL-cholesterol levels. This is of particular interest because olive oil is rich in monounsaturated fatty acids.

There is an inverse relationship between fish consumption and heart disease which may be related to the intake of the poly-unsaturated omega-3-fatty acids. These fatty acids reduce triglyceride but possibly exert their main effect by inhibiting thrombosis. Most other animal fats have the reverse effect. Not all vegetable oils are high in unsaturated fatty acids. The so-called 'tropical oils' such as palm oil and coconut oil are little dif-ferent from animal fats in this respect (see Table 5.2). They are very high in saturated fats and their inclusion in many processed foods such as biscuits and cakes or as cooking oils represents a hidden hazard. The label 'vegetable oil' is not a guarantee of sat-isfactory fatty-acid composition. Even oils which should be rich in polyunsaturated fatty acids may be affected by the process of manufacture. In general 'cold-pressed' oils are better than those where some heat extraction method has been used because repeated heating leads to a gradual hydrogenation turning polyunsaturated fatty acids into trans fatty acids. Major contribu-tors of trans fatty acids in the diet are margarine, baked, and fried foods. Both trans fatty acids and saturated fatty acids increase total and LDL cholesterol concentrations in blood. As yet, however, there is no conclusive evidence that trans fatty acid intake is a risk factor for coronary heart disease but it is recom-mended that trans fatty acid intake should not rise above the cur-rent 2% of energy intake.

Diet is not the only factor which influences levels of choles-terol fractions (Fig. 5.2). There appear to be hereditary factors which determine which individuals will increase their LDL-cholesterol levels on unfavourable diets, whereas others can cope with them with impunity. Exercise raises HDL and lowers total cholesterol. Smoking has the opposite effect and falls in HDL-cholesterol have been demonstrated in teenagers within a few months of commencing smoking. Certain types of person-ality seem to be associated with adverse blood cholesterol pat-terns. These additional factors have led at least some experts to doubt whether changing the dietary patterns of the whole population is the best way to tackle the problem of atheroscle-rosis, believing that attention should be concentrated on those most at risk.

Table 5.2. Fatty acid composition of commonly used foods

Food	Saturated (g/100 g food)	Monounsaturated (g/100 g food)	Polyunsaturated (g/100 g food)
High in MUFA			
Olive oil	14.0	69.3	11.2
Rapeseed oil*	5.3–6.6	57–64	25–32
Peanut oil	18.8	47.9	28.5
High in PUFA			
Margarine (PUFA)	19.1	15.9	60.2
Soya bean oil	14.0	24.3	56.7
Sunflower oil	13.1	31.8	50.0
Maize (corn) oil	16.4	29.3	49.3
Cottonseed oil	25.6	21.3	48.1
High in SFA			
Coconut oil	85.2	6.6	1.2
Suet	56.2	36.6	1.2
Butter	49.0	26.1	2.2
Palm oil	45.3	44.6	8.3
Lard	41.8	41.7	9.0

*There are two types of rapeseed oil—higher or lower in erucic acid and monounsaturates.
Key: MUFA—monounsaturated fatty acids; PUFA—polyunsaturated fatty acids; SFA—saturated fatty acids.

Some children are particularly at risk. Familial hypercholes-terolaemia is a relatively common genetic disorder in which lev-els of LDL-cholesterol are raised from early life and cholesterol lowering regimens are indicated from childhood. The underlying abnormality is a reduction of LDL receptors in the liver. Apart from this specific genetic condition, there is a range of blood lipids levels in the general population, which is partly genetically determined. These familial differences can be detected within what is generally regarded as the normal range.

Familial hypercholesterolaemia

Type IIa hyperlipidaemia is an autosomal dominant disorder resulting in elevation of the LDL-cholesterol lipid fraction from early life. It is associated with early coronary artery disease. As genetic diseases go it is common with about 1:500 individuals likely to be heterozygous for the condition. This means that 1:500 children are at risk of premature vascular disease, representing a serious public health problem. Because most heterozygotes reach the reproductive age, the chance of a couple both carrying the gene having children is 1:250 000. Thus about 1 in a million of the population will be homozygous with the very severe form of the disease. However, it is the heterozygous form which con-stitutes the really significant problem because it is relatively so common.

Screening children for CVD risk factors

There is good evidence that the onset of vascular disease can be prevented or delayed by lowering the blood cholesterol levels. Despite this there is little enthusiasm for screening programmes. One of the problems is that there is no test which can be used for screening populations that accurately predicts later cardio-vascular disease. An elevated blood cholesterol value in child-hood is only a risk factor for an elevated cholesterol as an adult, which in turn is a risk factor for heart disease. Some argue that screening would have negative effects including overuse of lipid lowering drugs, and the labelling of a large number of well chil-dren as having 'an illness'.

At present, identifying children is a random affair determined by the alertness of individual clinicians who identify a family history of early (<55 years) heart disease. Very few children are actually referred for dietary advice. All relatives of individuals with early-onset atherosclerosis should have serum lipid concentrations determined. In the first instance analysis of random blood lipids should be carried out. If these are within the normal range for age nothing further needs to be done, but they should be repeated periodically. If blood lipids are elevated, fasting concentrations must be determined. Continued elevation of LDL-cholesterol would warrant dietary treatment. The occasional borderline value should be followed up with a repeat test at six monthly intervals. The management of hypercholesterolaemia is discussed in Chapter 11.

Salt and hypertension

Populations with high average intakes of salt are likely to have higher average systolic blood pressures and salt intake appears to predict rise in blood pressure with age. Certain ethnic groups, Afro-Caribbean in particular, are at risk of hypertension. This may be because populations who originate from tropical climates have a tendency to retain salt as a protection against losses of sodium in sweat. Hypertension with stroke, rather than atherosclerosis with coronary disease, is the principle risk for black people in the United States. This appears to be related to the high sodium content of the diet. Similarly in Japan, the traditional fish diet which is high in salt also appears to increase the prevalence of hypertension despite a low incidence of atherosclerosis.

Whilst there is a growing scientific consensus that salt does increase blood pressure no targets for dietary salt restriction are given in *The health of the nation*, although in a report on nutrition and cardio-vascular disease a recommendation was made to reduce salt intake to 6 g (100 mmol soduim) daily together with an increase in potassium intake. Similar recommendations have been made in the United States and some other countries. Most dietary salt (65–85%) comes from processed foods and any attempt to limit intake would have considerable implications for manufacturers. Children and adolescents are major consumers of these foods, in particular snack foods. Not surprisingly industry has attempted to refute the unhealthy implications of adding salt to food, the cheapest way of making it more palatable. Despite these endeavours there is some evidence that the sodium content of food is slowly being reduced. This would seem to be an important step forward in attempts to reduce premature deaths from heart disease, but there is clearly much more progress to be made.

Diet and the general population

Policy-making in this field remains a thorny issue. Much depends on the view taken of the early origins of cardio-vascular disease. Whilst there is a clear case for placing all children with familial hypercholesterolaemia on a cholesterol-lowering diet with relatively high unsaturated fatty acid intake, greater controversy surrounds the point at which dietary intervention is appropriate to reduce the risk of disease in the general population. The COMA report *Nutritional aspects of cardiovascular disease* (see reference in further reading section) has made recommendations for all individuals over the age of 5 years. These recommendations cover a wide range and represent a prescription for healthy eating including:

- energy intake from fat should not exceed 35%
- unsaturated to saturated fatty acid ratio of at least 0.45
- avoid obesity
- increase fibre intake
- salt intake should not increase.

Their recommendations have to be seen in a wider context of lifestyle changes including not smoking (the most important single avoidable risk factor), more exercise, and avoidance of stress.

The reasons for excluding those under 5 from these recommendations was partly because of the uncertainty regarding the age of the onset of true atherosclerosis and the lack of convincing evidence that what happens in the young child is of critical importance. In the absence of compelling arguments, the concerns about the ill-effects of manipulation of lipid intake in the very young was given paramount importance. There remains a body of opinion which argues for the guidelines to be applied to children under 5 years. Some of the COMA recommendations are in fact uncontentious even in the under 5s. There is general agreement with the view that salt intake should not increase and that obesity should be avoided. The difficulty concerns the levels of fat and fibre which the very young should be allowed and the nature of the fat.

Undoubtedly, a gap exists in the recommendations for healthy eating between the ages of 6 months and 5 years. At the earlier age, most infants will still be receiving the bulk of their food intake either as breast milk or as infant formula. Thus approximately 50 % of caloric intake will come from fat. Thereafter, there is a progressive reduction in the amount of fat in the diet as solid foods replace milk but there are fears that the type of food eaten by many youngsters will be too high in animal fats. Furthermore if children obtain a substantial amount of their food in a deep fried form, for example fried fish and chips, even if the fat used is initially high in polyunsaturated fatty acids with repeated heating the fats will become hydrogenated and therefore higher in trans fatty acids.

Although great emphasis has been given to fats high in polyunsaturated fatty acids such as sunflower oil, there is increasing evidence that diets which contain oils with a high content of monounsaturated fatty acids such as olive oil are particularly protective. This may account for the apparent benefits of the 'Mediterranean diet'. The reason for this protective effect appears to be the increase in HDL-cholesterol which they engender.

It is probably desirable to continue with breast milk or infant formula until about one year of age. This will ensure that a high proportion of the fat intake will be low in saturated fatty acids. The current recommendation is that whole cows' milk be substituted after one year. If this is done it is not possible immediately to bring the proportion of energy as fat to the 35% recommended for the over 5s. Nor in the opinion of paediatric dietitians or most paediatricians is it desirable. The problem is that there is a conflict between the recommendation to reduce dietary fat and the fact that many toddlers depend on milk fat for a substantial part of their energy intake. While some households might be able to maintain adequate intake in young children fed skimmed or semi-skimmed milk there is a real danger that at least some children will become undernourished and deficient in fat soluble vitamins.

Thus the laudable aim of having similar foods for the whole family founders on the special needs of very young children. Some sort of compromise seems essential if the nutrition of all children is to be safeguarded. The change in fat intake from 50% of energy at 6 months to 35% at 5 years needs to be accomplished gradually, not by a rapid switch from formula or breast milk to skimmed or semi-skimmed milk but by a gradual reduction of the proportion of whole milk in the diet. At the same time it is desirable that any non-milk fat should be high in unsaturated fatty acids and especially include monounsaturated fatty acids.

In the United States it has been recommended that the fat intakes of children from 2 years of age should not exceed 30% of total energy. Some paediatricians, as in Britain, have urged caution since there is already evidence that such radical recommendations can lead to malnutrition. More recently Canada has changed its recommendations to include a statement that 'fat intake should not decrease to the recommended level until growth is complete'.

At two years of age semi-skimmed milk may be introduced provided the rest of the diet is properly balanced and the reduction in fat intake is not too drastic. Margarines high in unsaturated fats, and uncooked oils such as olive oil on salads should be used, and further encouragement of the British public to use these fats is desirable.

Similarly, the recommendation for an increase in dietary fibre must take into account the fact that at six months of age the diet is essentially fibre-free. After two years of age the fibre intake can gradually be increased (see Chapter 3).

Can children be programmed to poor eating habits?

There have been claims that if babies and young children become habituated to certain eating styles this may be perpetuated as a permanent tendency. Thus children given very sweet foods might develop a life-long preference for high sucrose foods. Similar ideas have been put forward for salt intake and overall energy consumption. The idea of the 'sweet tooth' conditioned by the nature of food intake prior to the presence of teeth has had wide currency. There is in fact an innate preference for sweet tasting food, probably because sweetness indicates bio- logical safety. There is no clear evidence to support the idea that giving babies very sweet food will habituate them to prefer such food for the rest of their lives. Introduction to a wide range of foods early in life may help to influence long-term eating habits. A very gradual introduction to a healthy COMA-style diet is to be recommended from weaning until these recommendations are achieved at around five years of age. The pattern set at one year of age should continue with a very gradual further reduction in fat and increase in fibre bearing in mind that it is always impor- tant to ensure that children have an adequate energy intake.

Principles of good eating

By 5 years of age the diet should contain no more than 35% of energy as fat with a balance between polyunsaturated, monoun- saturated, and saturated fatty acids. Opinions differ as to the exact ratios to be achieved but certainly saturated fatty acids should not exceed a ratio of 0.45; some would recommend a lower level. This implies restricting the amount of animal fat and vegetable oils high in saturated fatty acids such as palm and coconut oil. Excessive intake of polyunsaturated fatty acids should also be avoided and a judicious balance of intake of oils such as sunflower and soya which are very high in polyunsatu- rated fat and olive oil which is high in monounsaturated fats should be the aim. As we have already indicated we believe that between two and five years the transition should take place grad- ually, not so much in relation to the proportion of the various fatty acids but in total amount of fat as energy. For example while the two year old should continue to receive whole milk the rest of the fat intake should be moderated and comprise oils and fats high in mono- and polyunsaturated fats (Table 5.2). Convenience and other processed foods should be carefully scrutinized for the exact composition of their fat content.

Before weaning begins, the diet is essentially fibre-free. The weaning process itself introduces fibre. Foods which contain fibre suitable for children under one year of age are included in the weaning schedule in Chapter 2. Thereafter introduction of a wider variety of solid foods gradually increases naturally occurring fibre and should include foods which contain both soluble and insoluble fibre (Table 5.3). Pure fibre products such as wheat or oat bran should not be part of any child's normal diet.

It is desirable for children to have energy intakes that meet their needs without establishing patterns of excessive intake. Although, as we discuss in Chapter 10, caloric intake cannot be related directly to obesity in an individual child, there is no doubt that in societies where the overall energy intake is excessive an increased incidence of obesity results.

Table 5.3. Examples of foods high in fibre

Cereal Foods
Wholemeal and granary bread
Wholegrain breakfast cereals e.g. Weetabix, Shredded Wheat, Bran
  Flakes
Oats*, porridge*
Wholewheat pasta
Brown rice

Vegetables and Fruits
Vegetables—especially:
  legumes*/pulses*
  peas*
  beans*
fruits—all types including skin when edible

Nuts
Nuts—all types**
Peanut butter

---

  * Oats, beans, and pulse vegetables are particularly high in soluble fibre which may reduce blood cholesterol levels.
  ** Whole nuts should not be given to children under 5 years of age.

Snacks form an important part of the diets of young children and ensure that they do not fall short in their energy intake. However, they are a two edged sword as they can lead to an uncontrolled intake of energy. Many of the processed snack foods most popular with children are energy-dense and high in saturated fat, sugar, and salt. Thus while it is desirable for children to have some snacks, care is needed in what is offered. Some examples of suitable snacks are given in Table 3.2. It is important to remember that most soft drinks contain high concentrations of energy while being low in nutrients.

We have not given precise recommendations for amounts and nature of foods to be offered because of the great variation in the requirements of children, family preferences, ethnic differences, and the idiosyncratic eating patterns of young children. The availability of a wide range of foods within the general principles outlined should ensure a satisfactory intake.

The basis for healthy eating for children should incorporate the following:

- a wide variety of foods
- moderate intake of fats with emphasis on those high in monounsaturated and polyunsaturated fatty acids but low in saturated fatty acids
- the inclusion of high-fibre foods
- a minimal use of salt
- energy and protein intake to meet growth requirements
- adequate intake of vitamins and minerals.

The 'Barker hypothesis'

Professor David Barker and colleagues at the University of Southampton have generated a considerable amount of epidemiological research expanding the general theme that nutritional factors affecting the fetus and the young infant have long-lasting effects and are important causes of adult illness, such as coronary heart disease (CHD), stroke, and chronic bronchitis. They have postulated that early nutrition has decisive influences on subsequent metabolism and programme the development of risk factors such as raised blood pressure, fibrinogen concentration, factor VII concentration, and glucose intolerance, which are later determinants of CHD.

One intriguing paradox which stimulated early research in this area was that although CHD is an illness associated with affluent western societies, within the UK it is more common amongst the poorest sections of the population. This raised the possibility that there could be deprivation related factors at work which then predispose to the negative effects of 'affluence'. Comparisons of the present day prevalence of CHD in defined geographical areas with distribution of infant mortality during the early part of the century gave a fascinating clue. In areas in the north of England where CHD is common, infant mortality rates had been high, whereas in areas of the south-east where CHD is less common, infant mortality had been low. There have been a number of studies linking poor growth with an increased risk of CHD, and it seemed possible that adverse socio-economic conditions (including poor nutrition) acting on families and contributing to infant mortality might also exert long-term effects on those children who did not die but survived into adulthood.

An alternative explanation might be that people with poor living standards and inadequate nutrition in early life continue to live in a similar way such that later life-style influences are the determinants of disease. A study of three adjacent towns in Lancashire suggested that this was not the case. Early this century Nelson, Colne, and Burnley were all textile towns, but socio-economic conditions were worst in Burnley and best in Nelson. More recently, differences in socio-economic conditions between the three towns have largely disappeared, yet CHD rates are highest in Burnley and lowest in Nelson. This supports the view that adverse factors operating early rather than later in life have most to do with risk of CHD.

One of the ways of investigating the effects of early nutrition on adult health is to find places where detailed infant measurements were recorded early this century and then search out both the adult survivors and the cause of death in those who died. Such records were kept in Hertfordshire and showed that the death rate from CHD fell with increasing birth weight, and particularly with increasing weight at one year of age. These findings support the hypothesis that factors operating through the mother (determining birthweight) and health and nutrition in infancy (which influence growth in the first year of life) are both related to later risk of CHD.

Studies of surviving men still living in Hertfordshire with available data from infancy showed that those with lower birth weight and lower weight at one year were more likely as adults to have higher blood pressure and impaired glucose tolerance or diabetes. In addition, adult lung function was found to be impaired if either birth weight or weight gain during infancy had been low, or if there had been respiratory infection during infancy. Those who had been of lower weight at one year, when investigated as adults, also had higher plasma concentrations of apolipoprotein B and of the clotting factors fibrinogen and factor VII, all of which are associated with an increased risk of CHD. From these studies it seems clear that not only death rates from coronary heart disease but also many of the physiological variables which increase the risk of heart disease are adversely affected by impaired growth of the fetus or infant. Animal studies have indicated that this may be because influences which restrain growth during critical periods of early life permanently affect organ size and function.

The implications of this work are that good nutrition and a healthy environment during pregnancy and early childhood are likely to have long-term health gains. This does not negate the importance of attempting to alter risk factors (such as obesity) in later life, but suggests that a change in focus away from concentrating resources predominantly on persuading adults to adopt more 'healthy' life-styles may be important in terms of public health policy.

Iron deficiency

Iron deficiency is the most common single nutrient deficiency in the world affecting perhaps one billion people, with infants, children, and women most at risk. It is common even in industrialized countries like the UK and the USA, where some studies have found the prevalence in young children to be as high as 25%. About 10% of dietary iron is derived primarily from the haemoglobin and myoglobin of meat and is referred to as haem iron; it is readily absorbed. Non-haem iron is in the form of iron salts found in vegetable and plant protein foods, and accounts for about 90% of dietary iron; its absorption is highly variable. Ascorbic acid enhances the absorption of non-haem iron, as do meat, fish, and poultry. Inhibitors of absorption include bran, polyphenols, oxalates, phytates, vegetable fibre, tannins, and phosphates. Orange juice, which is high in vitamin C, taken with a meal doubles the absorption of non-haem iron, whereas tea, high in tannins, decreases it by 75%.

Breast milk and cows' milk both contain about 0.5–1.0 mg of iron per litre but, iron from breast milk is much better absorbed. The following are recommendations to prevent iron deficiency in infants:

• provide breast milk for five to six months
• if breast milk is unavailable use an iron fortified formula (12 mg/l)
• use an iron-fortified cereal amongst the earliest weaning foods
• avoid whole cows' milk during the first year of life because it may cause occult gastrointestinal bleeding.

In addition to anaemia, iron deficiency may also lead to impaired exercise capacity, changes in small bowel permeability, and possible increased risk of infection. Most importantly, there are considerable data indicating that iron deficiency is associated with impaired development during infancy, adverse effects on IQ and learning tasks in preschoolchildren, and poor educational achievement in those of school age. Of further concern is the intriguing evidence suggesting that maternal iron deficiency anaemia is linked to an increased risk to the child of hypertension in adult life.

Iron, together with calcium, vitamins A, D, and riboflavin is likely to be deficient in the diet of adolescents. In a national survey of diet in the UK among the 16–24 age group, convenience food, snacks, and confectionery predominated, with a notable shortage of fresh fruit and vegetables. In a recent study of 11–14 year olds, 11% of white and 22% of Indian girls in London were found to be anaemic. It was clear from this study that low haemoglobin is related to a complex interaction of different factors including dieting, early menarche, and social background. This suggests that devising effective interventions may be far from simple.

Bone disease

Rickets

Vitamin D is derived from the diet and the effect of ultraviolet light on the skin. Deficiency of vitamin D in the growing child leads to rickets, a metabolic disorder especially common during the Industrial Revolution because of poor nutrition and lack of exposure to sunlight. The introduction of vitamin D supplements under the Welfare Food Scheme in the early 1940s was associated in the following years with an almost complete abolition of nutritional rickets. In the 1960s and early 1970s rickets reappeared, among the Asian immigrant population of Britain. There is now evidence that rickets in this group has declined with adequate vitamin D supplementation.

Asian mothers with osteomalacia (vitamin D deficient bone disease) need vitamin D supplements during pregnancy and lactation if rickets is to be avoided in their offspring. Other nutritional disorders may coexist and in a Birmingham study of 145 Asian children, of the two fifths found to be anaemic half also had low plasma vitamin D, while another one fifth had low plasma vitamin D without anaemia. Dietary intake of vitamin D in the Asian community does not differ from that of non-immigrant groups, except among those who are vegetarian. The consumption of high-fibre cereal diets (including chapattis which contain phytate and fibre) is thought to be related to low vitamin D status, and limited exposure to sunlight remains an important factor.

The pathological effects of vitamin D deficiency include a failure to lay down mineral in the bony matrix together with expansion of cartilage tissue so that swelling occurs at the lower end of the radius and ulna, tibia and fibula. In young infants sitting, crawling and walking may be delayed and once weight bearing begins bowing of the legs or knock knees sometimes occurs. The skull bones may be soft (craniotabes) and examination of the chest sometimes reveals a 'rachitic rosary' due to enlargement of the costo-chondral junctions. In older children and adolescents the main symptoms may be pain on walking, or a waddling gait and deformity of the long bones. Clinical diagnosis is unreliable and most paediatricians rely on classical splaying and fraying of the end of the radius in the wrist X-ray. Ideally the diagnosis of primary nutritional vitamin D deficiency rickets is confirmed by healing of the lesion following modest doses of vitamin D, 10–50 μg daily, although sometimes several large doses (e.g. 5000 μg) are given to ensure compliance; this is known as stosstherapy. Premature infants are particularly at risk of bone disease and routinely need vitamin D supplements as well as sufficient mineral intake. The inclusion of foods rich in vitamin D is important from weaning onwards. Suitable foods include milk, eggs, oily fish, liver, fortified cereals, and margarine.

Osteoporosis

Osteoporosis (demineralization of normal bone) is a bone disorder which causes premature disability among many elderly people, particularly women. Although genetic factors are of considerable importance, the risk of bone damage and fractures from osteoporosis during later life are also related to the achievement of peak bone mass, which in turn is thought to be determined largely by dietary intake of calcium during growth. Studies in children have shown that dietary calcium supplementation does positively influence bone mineral density and with 40–50% of the skeletal mass deposited during adolescence, the impact of good dietary practice at this age may have considerable implications in later life. High impact physical exercise such as step aerobics is also another important contributory factor in building up bone mineral content which is strongly correlated with lean body mass.

Cancer

Although 23% of all deaths in Britain are from cancer, developments in treatment of malignant disease over the last twenty five years seem to have had little impact on overall mortality. Some have suggested that cancer should be viewed as a preventable condition rather than as a treatable disease, and the role of diet in influencing cancer risk is an area of considerable interest. There is mounting, but as yet inconclusive evidence that diets relatively low in meat and fat and high in vegetables, starchy staple foods, cereals, and fruits are associated with a lower occurrence of cancers of the stomach, large bowel, breast, ovary, and prostate.

Exactly how dietary risk factors operate is unclear, but complex genetic and environmental interactions are likely to apply in most cancers. One possibility is that there may be inherited or acquired differences in metabolic pathways that activate or inactivate dietary carcinogens and influence the risk of cancer. A high consumption of meat, for example, has been associated with an increased risk of colorectal cancer, possibly because cooking meat generates the production of amines which are capable of inducing tumours. Some individuals seem better at fuelling the chemical reaction which converts amines into mutagenic products (so called fast acetylators), and appear to be at increased risk of developing large bowel cancer.

One important area of research is to identify those nutritional factors which may serve to counteract the activities of substances ingested as part of our food which have the potential for damaging DNA and inducing malignant change in cells. For many years there has been a belief that fermented foods, particularly milk products, have beneficial health effects, and epidemiological studies have pointed to a protective effect of cultured dairy products against breast cancer.

The initiation of carcinogenesis is probably an irreversible chemical event which may then be promoted by chemicals which in themselves are not carcinogenic. Promotion is mediated by oxygen radicals and any food items which have been shown to have protective effects may do so because they are antioxidant; conversely, those which promote carcinogenesis may be responsible for an increase in the oxidant burden. Fruit and vegetables in particular, seem to have a protective effect against cancers and contain a wide variety of potentially anticarcinogenic substances. A high intake of raw tomatoes, for example, was found to be associated with a decreased risk of gastrointestinal malignancy; tomatoes contain large quantities of lycopene, a hydrocarbon carotenoid and powerful antioxidant.

The antioxidant protection offered by vitamins C, E, and the carotenoids may only be derived from their consumption in complex mixtures with other compounds in foods rather than as vitamin supplements. It would appear therefore that the general healthy eating recommendations to increase fruit and vegetable consumption to a minimum of five servings daily may, along with other dietary changes offer some protection against certain cancers.

Further reading

Auket, M.A., Parks, Y.A., Scott, P.H., and Wharton, B.A. (1986). Treatment with iron increases weight gain and psychomotor development. *Archives of Disease in Childhood*, **61**, 849–57.

Barker, D.J.P. (1997). Fetal nutrition and cardiovascular disease in later life. *British Medical Bulletin*, **53**, (1), 96–108.

Canadian Paediatric Society, Health Canada (1995). Nutrition recommendations update: Dietary fats and children. *Nutrition Reviews*, **53**, (12), 367–75.

Department of Health (1994). *Nutrition aspects of cardiovascular disease*. Report on health and social subjects, No. 46. HMSO, London.

Godlee, F. (1996). The food industry fights for salt. *British Medical Journal*, **312**, 1239–40.

HMSO (1994). *The health of the nation*. A consultative document for health in England. HMSO, London.

James, J., Brown, J., Douglas, M., Cox, J., and Stocker, S. (1992). Improving the diet of under fives in a deprived inner city practice. *Health Trends*, **24**, 161–4.

Lifshitz, F. and Tarim, O. (1996). Considerations about dietary fat restrictions for children. *Journal of Nutrition*, **126**, (4), 1031S–41S.

Paneth, N. and Susser, M. (1995). Early origin of coronary heart disease (the Barker hypothesis). *British Medical Journal*, **310**, 411–12.

Steinmetz, K.A. and Potter, J. (1996). Vegetables, fruit, and cancer prevention: A review. *Journal of the American Dietetic Association*, **96**, 1027–39.

Willett, W.C., Sacks, F., Trichopoulou, A., Drescher, G., Ferro-Luzzi, A., Helsing, E., and Trichopoulos, D. (1995). Mediterranean diet pyramid: a cultural model for healthy eating. *American Journal of Clinical Nutrition*, **61**, 1402S–6S.

6

....

Cultural and ethnic diets

Many ethnic groups have from time immemorial adapted their food intake according to religious practice or to the availability of certain foods. As a result they have developed cuisines which are both aesthetically satisfying and nutritionally adequate. There is evidence that some ethnic groups have developed evolutionary adaptations to cope with what for others might be diets deficient in certain nutrients. Problems can arise when people adopt some of the eating habits of a different culture or ethnic group. Children in particular may develop nutritional deficiencies as a consequence. For these reasons anyone wishing to change their eating habits drastically should seek dietary advice.

Difficulties also occur when people used to a particular range of foods and certain climatic conditions find themselves in an environment very different from that of their homelands. For example children from the Indian subcontinent living in rural conditions in their homelands usually obtain sufficient vitamin D because of the amount of ultraviolet light to which they are exposed, despite low levels of vitamin D in the diet. The same diet may lead to deficiency in those parts of the world with less sunlight. Advice may be required on how to adapt their traditional cooking and eating habits in order to achieve a good balance of nutrients and in some cases dietary supplementation during infancy, childhood, and pregnancy may be required.

When families move to a new country they bring with them their dietary customs; however, over time these become influenced by the food habits of the indigenous population and lead to many individual variations. We have given some of the general dietary guidelines for various ethnic and cultural groups but it is important to remember that there will be many individual variations within these groups.

Vegetarian diets

This general term describes all diets in which the amount and character of animal foods ingested is limited. Approximately 5% of the UK population claim to be vegetarian and the number may well be greater than this. With the promotion of healthy eating recommendations more people may well adopt vegetarian diets. People choose to follow a vegetarian diet for a number of reasons including ethical and ecological concerns and beliefs in the health promoting properties of the diet.

Vegetarian diets vary considerably in the extent to which they exclude animal products. The more meat and animal products are excluded, the greater the potential risk, particularly to children, of diets which are not carefully planned. In principle the problem to be borne in mind is that vegetables have a lower concentration of proteins than meat or dairy products, and that the ratio of essential amino acids is also lower than that of animal proteins. Thus greater volumes of protein containing foods have to be consumed. This can cause nutritional compromise in small children if the diet is not carefully balanced to ensure adequate intake of all nutrients. Vegetables are also inherently less well supplied with certain nutrients, particularly fat-soluble vitamins. The very high fibre intake which accompanies the predominantly vegetable diet may cause problems in younger children because:

• fibre reduces the availability of some nutrients
• it is bulky and very filling

• it leads to an inadequate energy intake
• fibre can cause toddler diarrhoea

These problems can be overcome with careful, age appropriate planning and preparation of the diet. On the other hand a predominantly vegetable diet ensures a healthier intake of unsaturated fatty acids and an adequate intake of fibre and other beneficial nutrients found in vegetables and fruits. Vegetarians as a group have been seen to have a lower incidence of some chronic diseases such as heart disease and some cancers and less hypertension, obesity, and non-insulin-dependent diabetes.

A vegetarian can be defined as 'one who lives wholly or principally on vegetable foods; a person who on principle, abstains from any form of animal food or at least such as is obtained by the destruction of life' (Oxford English Dictionary). It is usual to classify vegetarian diets according to their degree of restriction of animal products, in ascending order of restriction these are;

1. Partial vegetarians   This category includes all those groups who exclude some, but not all, animal products. For example some exclude red meat but will eat poultry or fish. Partial vegetarians should have little or no problem in providing a balanced diet for their children. Problems may arise if the child eats the low protein vegetables and potatoes but refuses the food provided as a substitute for meat or if milk is not included. The nutrients most likely to be deficient in this group are iron and protein and this is particularly likely if foods are excluded from the diet and not replaced, for example the child who leaves the meat portion and eats only the potatoes and vegetables.

2. Lacto-ovo-vegetarians   Lacto–ovo-vegetarians avoid all meat, meat products, poultry, and fish. They include milk, milk products, and eggs in the diet and should also include a wide variety of vegetables, cereals, beans, and pulses. Nutrient deficiencies are unlikely in this group; however intakes of some nutrients may be low.

3. Lacto-vegetarians   Lacto-vegetarians avoid all meat, meat products, poultry, fish, and eggs. They do, however eat milk

products and drink milk. The diet should contain generous quantities of high-protein vegetables such as beans, nuts, and pulses in addition to a variety of other vegetables, cereals, milk, and milk products.

4. Vegans   Vegans exclude all animal products from their diets including additives such as rennet and cholecalciferol which may be incorporated into manufactured products. A vegan diet is usually part of a philosophy of life and can be part of a very healthy life-style but the diets, particularly of young children, pregnant, and lactating women must be carefully planned to ensure adequate nutrition and avoid serious vitamin and mineral deficiencies. Deficiencies of protein, energy, vitamin B_{12}, calcium, zinc, and fat soluble vitamins have all been described with poorly planned diets, both in breast-fed babies and young children.

If an adult or child becomes a 'new vegetarian' it is important that they do not simply exclude animal products from their diets. The foods excluded must be replaced by others (Table 6.1), such as pulses, nuts, seeds, and cereal foods thus providing necessary protein, vitamins, and minerals. Table 6.2 lists some food sources of various 'at risk' nutrients.

Feeding vegetarian children

It is important to be aware of the fact that children require a higher intake of nutrients in relation to their body size than adults and this should be taken into account in planning vegetarian diets for the young.

Most vegetarians breast-feed their infants and continue breast-feeding well after the introduction of solid foods. This helps to ensure an adequate intake of essential nutrients provided that the mother's diet is satisfactory. In particular, essential amino acids are supplemented as well as vitamins and calcium. It is important to ensure that the maternal diet contains vitamin B_{12} especially if she is a vegan. Breast milk from vegan mothers is known to be low or deficient in B_{12} and supplementation of the mothers diet is recommended. A B_{12} supplement may also be required for the infant.

Table 6.1. Characteristics of vegetarian diets

Group	Foods excluded	Possible nutrient deficiencies	Suitable food substitutes
Partial vegetarian	red meats: beef, pork, lamb meat products offal	iron	poultry, fish, eggs, milk, cheese, yoghurt, beans, lentils, nuts, seeds
Lacto–ovo vegetarian	meat, fish, poultry	iron, zinc, vitamin B_6	eggs, milk, cheese, yoghurt, beans lentils, nuts, seeds
Lacto vegetarian	meat fish poultry eggs	iron, zinc, vitamins D, B_6	milk, cheese, yoghurt, beans, lentils, nuts, seeds
Vegan	meat fish poultry eggs milk yoghurt cheese	protein, energy, iron, calcium, zinc, vitamins, D, B_6, B_{12}	beans, lentils, nuts, seeds soya milk* rice milk*

*Fortified with calcium.

If the infant is bottle-fed an approved infant formula should be used. Cows' milk, goat's milk, and some soya preparations are not suitable as infant feeds. Table 6.3 lists the names of some of the breast milk substitutes which are used by vegetarian mothers and indicates which are suitable and which are potentially dangerous. It is important to remember that infant formulas may contain animal fats and therefore be unacceptable to vegetarians.

Infants of vegan parents can be fed on soya preparations which are approved infant formulas. There are a number of appropriate feeds now available (Table 6.3). Homemade soya 'milks' or liquid soya 'milk' purchased from health food shops

Table 6.2. Vegan food sources for selected 'at risk' nutrients

Iron	wholegrain cereals and breads
	fortified cereals
	dark green leafy vegetables
	beans, lentils and split peas
	dried fruits, nuts*
	tofu, quorn
	molasses, cocoa, curry powder
Calcium	fortified soya milk
	green leafy vegetables
	sunflower seeds*, sesame seeds
	almonds*, cashew nuts*
	legumes
Zinc	legumes and beans
	nuts*
	whole grains, wheat germ
Vitamin D	fortified margarine, fortified soya milk
	fortified cereals
	sunlight
Vitamin B_6	green leafy vegetables
	legumes and whole grains
Vitamin B_{12}	fortified soya milk, tofu
	yeast extracts
	Tastex, Barmene, Grape Nuts

*Whole nuts should not be given to children under 5 years of age.

should not be used as infant feeds as they do not contain adequate energy, vitamins, or minerals.

Goats' milk and ewes' milk are also not suitable feeds for babies because they:

• have a high solute load
• are low in folic acid

Table 6.3. Milk substitutes used by vegetarians and their suitability for infant feeding

Nutritionally complete (suitable for infants)	Nutritionally incomplete (not suitable for infants under one year of age)
Human breast milk*	
Milk based	
Cow and Gate Premium	cows' milk
Cow and Gate Plus	goats' milk
Farley's First Milk	ewes' milk
Farley's Second Milk	
Aptamil	
Milumil	
Soya based	
Isomil*	Liquid soya milk*
Prosobee*	Liquid rice milk*
InfaSoy	
OsterSoy*	
Wysoy*	

*Denotes suitability for vegans.

- are low in vitamins A, D, and C
- risk bacterial contamination if unpasteurized e.g. brucellosis and salmonella.

The vegetarian infant should be introduced to solids at the same time as non-vegetarian babies i.e. between 4–6 months and a weaning schedule is outlined in Table 6.4. Suitable first weaning foods include baby rice, smooth puréed vegetables or fruit (no added salt or sugar). Some proprietary weaning foods are suitable for vegetarians and fewer for vegans; many manufacturers indicate if the product is suitable for vegetarians. The baby should continue to be fed the full quantity of breast or formula feeds and solids should be gradually increased, introducing new tastes and textures. Care should be taken to use energy rich foods, especially as the child consumes less milk. This can be

Table 6.4. Suggested weaning foods for vegetarian babies

4–5 months		baby rice cereal*
		puréed cooked fruits
		puréed cooked vegetables
5–7 months	Add:	Weetabix, rusk*, and other cereals*
		vegetable and lentil or bean purées
		lentil and cereal purées
		milk puddings or custards**
		soya milk puddings and custards
7–12 months		Introduce thicker textures and lumps to the above foods.
	Add:	wholegrains, breads, pasta, and rice
		finely ground nuts
		chopped dried fruits
		cheese, eggs (if appropriate)
		tofu and quorn

*use milk free varieties for vegetarians.
**suitable for vegetarians but not vegans.

ensured by mixing breast milk or formula with solid foods. A mixture of cereals and pulses can be introduced gradually; however, care must be taken not to give the young child too much fibre. Beans and lentils should be well cooked and sieved initially. Beans which are partially cooked or raw may contain toxins such as trypsin inhibitors and haemaglutinins which can cause diarrhoea and vomiting. These are destroyed by boiling for at least ten minutes and it is important to note that slow cookers will not destroy the toxins.

Finely ground nuts and smooth nut butters may be introduced, but it should be remembered that they are potential food allergens and it may be wise to introduce them later rather than earlier (see Chapter 9). Whole nuts should not be offered before the age of five years and then only with caution because of the danger of inhalation. Proprietary baby foods have the advantage of being fortified with vitamins and minerals and the inclusion of at least one fortified cereal food is to be recommended. Vitamin drops should be given from one month to five years of age. In younger infants (1 month to 6 months) who are fed adequate volumes of formula vitamin drops are not required until the usual 6 months of age. In vegan babies it is essential to provide extra vitamin B_{12}, this is added to soya infant formulas, however breast fed babies may need supplements. Older children may be given Tastex, Barmene and yeast extracts which are rich in Vitamin B_{12}, unfortunately as these products are high in sodium they are unsuitable for infants. Grape nuts, fortified soya milks and tofu are also high in vitamin B_{12}.

The nutritional difficulties which are associated with vegetarian diets and which increase with degree of restriction of animal foods, arise from the fact that the diet is inevitably bulky and this may lead to undernutrition. Although vegan children appear to grow and develop within the normal range, they do tend to be lighter and leaner than the general population. It is therefore important to avoid the pitfalls of a bulky diet and to choose nutrient dense foods. Breast feeding or an approved infant formula should be continued as long as possible well past the weaning phase and at least until one year of age. One pint (500 ml) of full fat cows' milk or soya formula per day is desirable until two years of age to ensure a good source of energy, vitamins and minerals.

As the child gets older the problem of bulk declines making it possible to join fully with the normal family meals. A food group guide which includes suggested servings is given in Table 6.5. Growth should be monitored regularly and if poor growth is noted the first step should be to ensure that the child's diet is nutritionally adequate.

Cult diets

Other vegetarian diets, sometimes classified as cult diets, include macrobiotic diets such as the Zen macrobiotic diet and fruitarian diets. Many of these diets are essentially vegetarian and have the same nutritional cautions we have already discussed; however, some are much more restrictive and exclude many foods making a nutritionally balanced intake impossible, particularly in children.

Table 6.5. Daily food guide for vegetarian children

Food group	Serving size	Number of servings		
		1–4 years	4–6 years	6 years–adolescence
Bread and rolls				
Preferably wholegrain	1 slice or roll	3	4	4–5
Cereals				
Wheat flour, bulgar wheat, wheat germ, rice, oatmeal, pasta, breakfast cereal	1–5 level tablespoons	1	2	2–3
Vegetables and fruits				
Citrus: oranges, orange juice, grapefruit, tangerines, satsumas	4–8 level tablespoons 60–120 ml juice	2	2	2
Dark green or orange: broccoli, spinach, kale, spring greens, watercress, carrots, dried apricots	4–6 level tablespoons	½	1	2–3
Other vegetables and fruits: potato, tomato, apple, banana, raisins, sweetcorn, avocado	4–6 level tablespoons	3	4	5–7

Table 6.5. (*Continued*)

Protein foods				
A variety daily				
Pulses: lentils, soya, kidney and other beans, split peas, tofu, tempeh, peanuts, peanut butter	pulses: 2–6 level tablespoons	3	3	3–4
Nuts and seeds: sunflower, sesame, pumpkin seeds; tahini; all nuts except coconut	nuts and seeds: 1–3 level tablespoons			
(Eggs, cheese for lacto–ovo vegetarians)				
Milk				
Fortified soya milk (cows' milk, yoghurt for lacto–ovo vegetarians)	250 ml	3	3	3–4
Fats				
Vegetable oil and margarine, preferably rapeseed, soya, olive (butter, ghee for lacto–ovo vegetarians)	1 level teaspoon	3	4	5
Other foods				
yeast extract (B_{12} fortified)	level tablespoon	1	1	1
black treacle	level tablesppon	1	1	1

Manual of dietetic practice, second edition (1994). Edited by Briony Thomas. Blackwell Science. Adapted from T.342 p. 322: *Daily food guide for vegitarian children and adults.*

Zen macrobiotic diets

Macrobiotics is a regimen based on 'keeping a balance between the Yin and Yang aspects of life' thus achieving optimal spiritual, mental, and physical development. Foods are divided into Yin and Yang and the goal is attained by working through ten levels of diet, gradually eliminating all animal products, and many fruits and vegetables. The final diet consists almost entirely of cereal (usually brown rice). Fluids may also be restricted.

In its early stages, the diet is not generally nutritionally deficient, but during the later stages serious inadequacies leading to deficiency can be produced. During infancy, the baby may be protected by breast-feeding but if breast milk is unavailable the macrobiotic regimen recommends a homemade grain and seed 'milk' which is totally unsuitable as an infant feed and will lead to malnutrition. Similar problems will arise on weaning the breast-fed baby onto a macrobiotic regimen and there have been a number of reports of harmful effects, including severe failure to thrive and malnutrition.

Fruitarians

Fruitarian diets are based on fruit and fermented, cooked cereals and seeds. Only produce harvested by means which do not damage the plant are eaten. These diets will also produce malnutrition and deficiency disorders in children.

Neither the Zen macrobiotic regimen nor the fruitarian diets can be safely adapted for young children. To give children such diets places their health and development at risk. In cases where parents insist on so doing, child-protection measures should be invoked. A compromise based on discussion and persuasion will usually result in the devising of a nutrition plan which is acceptable to the parents and is consistent with the child's well-being.

Obsession with 'healthy eating'

As has been discussed in Chapters 3 and 5, the current concern to protect children from the hazards of diet induced atherosclerosis is not without problems. In some cases the concern may become obsessional, leading to diarrhoea, fat-soluble vitamin deficiencies, and significant undernutrition. This results from the drastic restriction of fat intake and excessive provision of high fibre foods sometimes characterized as the 'muesli-belt syndrome'. Several reports in the literature have highlighted this danger, children following unsupervised, severely fat restricted diets have been seen to present with failure to thrive and malnutrition. All children on fat restricted diets should be followed by a paediatric dietitian to ensure a nutritionally adequate diet and normal growth.

Diets of different ethnic origins

The United Kingdom is home for many peoples who have migrated over the years from all parts of the world. They have naturally brought their traditional forms of cuisine with them as food and eating customs form a major part of cultural heritage and tradition. In their new surroundings these customs may result in nutritional problems, particularly in children. We outline here the major ethnic dietary variants which may be encountered. Most of the groups are Asian and embrace a number of religions, each with its own pattern of food restrictions. The most important are Hinduism, Islam (Moslems), Jainism, and Sikhism. Other major groups in the UK include the Afro-Caribbean population, a small number of whom are Rastafarians, and the various Chinese populations.

Asian diets

Approximately 30% of the Asian population in the UK are Hindu, most from the Gujarat region of India. Hinduism has at its core the idea that the soul is eternal and a belief in reincarnation. Hindus do not eat beef as the cow is considered sacred and usually do not eat pork. Some will eat other meats and fish although many are vegetarian and the more orthodox (women particularly) may not eat eggs. Hindus rely on pulses and dairy products for their proteins and wheat is their main staple in the form of chapattis, puris, and parathas. Ghee and oil are used in cooking. Possible nutritional deficiencies are similar to those outlined for vegetarians.

Jainism is an offshoot of Hinduism with similar beliefs and ideas. Most Jains, particularly women, are strict vegetarians and may refuse food which has been cooked in a utensil previously used for cooking meat. Many Jains also avoid what are described as 'hot' foods (lentils, carrots, onions, aubergines, chilli, ginger, dates, eggs, tea, honey, and brown sugar).

Moslems make up about 30% of the Asian population and follow the dietary laws laid down in the Koran. They are forbidden to eat pork or any product of the pig, or to eat the blood of any animal. Animals must be slaughtered according to the regulations and a short prayer said to render the meat 'halal'. Foods containing non-halal meats are forbidden. Only fish with fins or scales may be eaten. Alcohol is forbidden. Wheat, in the form of chapattis is the usual staple for Moslems from Pakistan and rice for those from Bangladesh.

Sikhs make up the other large group of the Asian population in the UK and have the fewest dietary restrictions. Most will not eat pork or beef but will eat lamb, poultry, eggs, and dairy produce. Some Sikhs are lacto–ovo-vegetarian. Wheat and rice are the main staples in the diet. Alcohol is not permitted.

Fasting plays a role in the religious life of all groups; however, young children and pregnant women are not normally expected to fast. Young children are strongly influenced by family food habits and there is a danger of weight loss if the child follows the adult pattern of fasting. It is important to remind parents that their children need to eat during these periods.

The lacto-vegetarian diet common to many Asians is potentially rachitogenic in Britain and in the 1970s some Asian children were noted to have florid or sub-clinical rickets. This is probably the combination of several factors, including low maternal vitamin D intake, low levels of vitamin D in breast milk as a consequence, a low intake of dietary vitamin D, and possibly a high intake of phytate-containing foods which inhibit the absorption of calcium and vitamin D. Late weaning onto a diet low in vitamin D may cause deficiency in later childhood. In the homelands this deficiency is compensated by the synthesis of vitamin D in the skin under the action of ultraviolet light of the sun. The relative lack of sunlight in Britain and the skin pigmentation of Asian children is probably the main limiting factor. Additionally there is tendency to late weaning and prolonged breast-feeding which may limit vitamin D intake. Vitamin D supplementation for Asian children is recommended from one month of age until five years of age. With more widespread vitamin D supplementation the incidence of rickets in this population has now greatly declined. The practice of supplementation with vitamin D should continue.

Weaning should be encouraged between the ages of 4–6 months using adapted family foods to avoid the problem of proprietary baby foods containing non-halal meat products. There is a tendency for Asian Moslem babies to be kept on milk-based food for too long and this may result in iron deficiency and can be aggravated by the use of cows' milk before one year of age. This practice is partly traditional and partly a result of anxieties about the religious acceptability of proprietary baby foods. Certain weaning foods are suitable and parents should be encouraged to seek them out and use them. They are supplemented with iron and should be encouraged in addition to other acceptable iron containing foods, for example egg yolk, halal beef or lamb (puréed if necessary), and green vegetables. It is also important to encourage foods which aid iron absorption i.e. those which are high in vitamin C.

Progression onto the normal family diet by approximately one year is desirable. Much support and advice may be necessary and the language gap may compound the difficulties of getting acceptance of these different feeding practices.

Afro-Caribbean diets

The Afro-Caribbean group is one of the largest ethnic minority groups in the UK. Many dietary practices have been adopted by this group and may include the use of traditional foods such as plantain, yam, and sweet potato. The starchy foods are generally served with small amounts of meat or fish and green leafy vegetables seasoned with herbs and spices. There are no major nutritional concerns provided a balanced diet is consumed.

Rastafarians

Rastafarians, a small subgroup within the Afro-Caribbean population, usually exclude all meat, fish, and preserved foods from their diets. Some are strict vegans while others will drink milk; eggs are often avoided and salt and alcohol are not taken. Areas of nutritional concern are in pregnant and lactating women and in young children. Late weaning onto highly starchy foods is common practice and there have been reports of iron deficiency anaemia and rickets in Rastafarian children. Those who follow a strict vegan diet may become deficient in vitamin B_{12} and folic acid particularly if intake of green vegetables is low.

Lactose intolerance

This phenomenon develops in large numbers of children of Asian and Afro-Caribbean origin who are genetically programmed to have falling levels of mucosal lactase after infancy. Tolerance of lactose is extremely variable. Lactose intolerance is discussed in Chapter 9.

Other ethnic groups

Orthodox Jews exclude pork, rabbit, shellfish, and eels from their diet. Meat must be ritually slaughtered and milk and its products not taken at the same meal as meat, following the biblical proscription against 'seething the kid in its mother's milk'.

The Chinese have few or no dietary restrictions. Pork is not eaten by the Chinese Moslem population. Wide varieties of foods are eaten and the emphasis varies from region to region. The main areas for concern are the high salt content of the traditional diet and the high fat and sugar consumption adopted, particularly by the younger generation, as they consume more Western convenience and fast foods.

In common with these ethnic groups, the diets of Poles, Italians, Greek, and Turkish Cypriots do not generally create nutritional problems or deficiencies in their children. As we have noted, the 'Mediterranean diet' may be near the ideal (Chapter 5).

It is important to bear in mind that not all members of ethnic groups follow the dietary restrictions equally and care should be taken to elucidate the precise nature of the diet and not to take it for granted.

Further reading

British Dietetic Association (1995). *Vegetarian diets: a position paper.* British Dietetic Association, Birmingham.

British Nutrition Foundation (1995). *Vegetarianism: briefing paper.* British Nutrition Foundation, London.

Dagnelie, P.C., van Stavern, W.A., Verschuren, S.A., and Hautuast, J.G. (1989). Nutritional status of infants aged 4–18 months on macrobiotic diets and matched omnivorous control infants: A population based mixed longitudinal study. 1: Weaning patterns, energy and nutrient intake: *European Journal of Clinical Nutrition*, **43**, 311–23.

Duggan, M.B. and Harbottle, L. (1996). The growth and nutritional status of healthy Asian children aged 4–40 months living in Sheffield. *British Journal of Nutrition*, **76**, 183–97.

Nathan, I., Hackett, A.F., and Kirby, S. (1996). The dietary intake of a group of vegetarian children aged 7–11 years compared with matched omnivores. *British Journal of Nutrition*, **75**, 533–44.

Sanders, T.A.B. and Manning, J. (1992). The growth and development of vegan children. *Journal of Human Nutrition and Dietetics*, **5**, 11–21.

....

7

Feeding problems in infants

A wide range of symptoms occur in young babies, associated with or ascribed to feeding or digestive processes. For the most part they are not due to serious organic disease and are not amenable to 'medical' treatment. Yet they are a cause of concern to parents and unfortunately can lead to emotional disturbance and distort the normal, parent–child relationship. They are also a happy hunting ground for theorists, unqualified 'experts', and quacks who exploit parents real anxieties either for financial gain or in order to further their own reputations. As a consequence there is much misdiagnosis of 'organic' cause and inappropriate investigation and treatment.

Growth assessment is an important component of evaluating the severity of feeding problems and growth failure is an indication for referral to a paediatrician.

Failure to thrive in breast-fed babies

Breast milk as the exclusive means of feeding infants remains the ideal. Nevertheless, there are circumstances in which the amount of milk produced by the mother may be insufficient for the needs of the infants. Beyond six months of age exclusive breast-feeding can lead to nutritional deficiencies, in particular iron deficiency and the natural progression is therefore to include some solid foods at this age.

More serious is the occasional infant who fails to thrive because inadequate food supply is unrecognized. Characteristically these babies become apathetic and quiet whilst appearing to be content; gross failure to thrive and dehydration can result. The diagnosis may sometimes be rejected by an often tired, depressed, and distraught mother deeply committed to breast-feeding and unwilling to accept 'failure'. The emotional reaction can be severe and great care must be taken not to aggravate tension. However, it is essential, to ensure that the baby gets extra feeds, although breast-feeding should continue.

In these situations intervention will include:

* regular weighing
* frequent breast-feeds on demand, with emphasis on correct technique
* complementary formula feeds given *after* breast-feed
* introduction of solids, if age appropriate
* emotional support for the mother.

Delay in establishment of breast milk supply

Occasionally, in a well-motivated mother, the breast-milk supply may fail to increase at an appropriate rate. The most usual cause of this is failure of the baby adequately to stimulate milk production by sucking. This in turn is most likely to occur if the baby is insufficiently hungry or not positioned correctly (see Chapter 2) when put to the breast. In some instances psychological factors may be at work which inhibit the various endocrine mechanisms already outlined. In such cases it will be apparent from plotting on centile charts, that the baby is going to lose more than 10% of its birthweight before it begins to gain. In these circumstances, judicious use of complementary feeding, combined with emotional support for the mother should tide the baby over until the milk supply is properly established. The essential factor to bear in mind is that the baby should still be hungry when put to the breast.

Jaundice

All normal infants have some degree of clinical or biochemical jaundice during the first few days of life. This is thought to be due to the immaturity of the liver enzyme glucuronyl transferase, which is necessary for the excretion of bilirubin. This so-called 'physiological' jaundice usually reaches a peak around day four of life and is almost never significant in healthy fullterm infants, but can require treatment with increased fluids and phototherapy particularly in the sick, premature infant.

In some infants jaundice persists for several weeks. In the overwhelming majority of infants it clears up with no further problems, but persisting jaundice beyond two weeks requires referral to a paediatrician for exclusion of serious disease such as biliary atresia.

Breast-fed infants are more likely to become jaundiced than formula-fed babies. Breast milk appears to contain a factor which inhibits the transferase enzyme, although the exact mechanism remains obscure. While stopping breast-feeding for several days leads to a diagnostic fall in bilirubin, this course of action is likely to cause failure of breast-feeding. Babies who develop mild physiological jaundice during the first week do not need to be offered supplementary feeds or additional drinks of water as these do not appear to change the course of the jaundice and may, in fact interfere with the establishment of breast-feeding. A final diagnosis of 'breast milk jaundice' should not be made unless other causes of persistent jaundice have been excluded.

Fears about 'hypoglycaemia'

Another reason often cited for supplementary feeding while the breast milk is coming in, is concern that the baby might develop hypoglycaemia as a consequence of starvation. This concern arose from the discovery that babies who are underweight at birth are likely to develop hypoglycaemia if fasted and such infants need to be fed adequately soon after birth. They have special problems because they have suffered intra-uterine malnutrition and so have reduced stores of glycogen in the liver and less fat than normal. This does not apply to fullterm, healthy infants whose livers contain glycogen and who can mobilize their fat stores to meet energy requirements. Provided the baby is being fed whenever it is hungry and is not losing weight excessively, breast-feeding should proceed without supplementation.

Breast-feeding problems

Failure to establish the milk supply may result, in a small number of women, from retraction of the nipple making it difficult for the baby to attach. In the first instance this may cause engorgement but eventually lactation failure will supervene. Good positioning is likely to be the most helpful intervention in this situation (see Chapter 2).

Engorgement may result from infrequent attempts to feed or putting the baby to the breast when not hungry (Fig. 7.1). A vicious cycle may then commence, with the nipple becoming more difficult to grasp, the pain making it more difficult for the mother to tolerate the sucking, and further trauma resulting from the infant's increasingly frustrated efforts to obtain milk, leading to cracking of the nipple and eventual infection. All this is mostly avoidable if care is taken with the initial phase of establishing lactation.

In addition to good positioning and frequent feeding, other helpful measures may include:

- placing a warm damp towel on the breast before feeding or having a warm shower
- cold compresses between feeding to help with pain
- gently expressing some milk to alleviate engorgement immediately prior to feeding
- use of analgesics (see Chapter 2 for safe drugs), if necessary, to minimize pain.

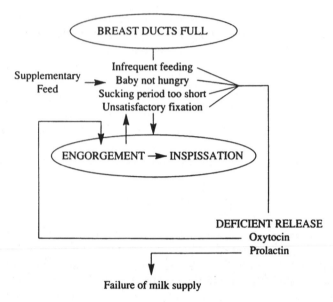

Fig. 7.1. Factors leading to breast engorgement and failure of milk supply.

Running out of milk

A common reason for stopping breast feeding is the belief that the milk has 'dried up'. There does seem to be a relative dip in milk production after a few weeks in some cases resulting in an increased demand by the baby to be fed. This can often be easily overcome by increasing stimulation by suckling the baby more frequently, ensuring that the mother is getting enough rest and that she has an adequate fluid intake. About 25% of infants who appear to be well established on the breast, being demand fed, at about 6−8 weeks of age require to be fed more frequently. The mother will find that during the day particularly, she may have to feed the baby as often as hourly; often these babies continue to sleep well at night. This can impose a strain on the mother leading to cessation of breast-feeding.

Unfortunately this can be interpreted by both mother and health adviser as evidence of 'running out of milk' whereas in fact it represents a short term re-adjustment. The baby, may indeed, at this point not be getting enough milk and responds in an entirely appropriate way, by demanding to be fed more often. The appropriate parental response should be to do just that—to feed the baby more frequently. This will quite rapidly lead to further stimulation and increase the supply of milk; usually within a few days the baby will settle back to a more usual routine. If this is carefully explained to the mother, she will be willing to accept a more frequent rate of feeding for a limited period—usually less than a week. Offering the baby supplementary feeds will almost certainly result in a reduction of milk supply, further unhappiness from the baby and eventual cessation of breast-feeding.

The 4–6 week period is often a low point for the mother of a young baby. The initial excitement will have worn off and the drudgery involved in the daily care of the infant may result in increasing tiredness. Parents are keen to renew their social and other activities, all of which may contribute to a degree of exhaustion. If this is coupled with an inadequate calorie and nutrient intake it may reflect in either a reduction of milk supply or a failure to increase it in line with the needs of the baby. Continued emotional support coupled with practical help from father or other family members to reduce the sheer physical demands, together with sensible dietary advice, may prevent many cases of secondary lactation failure.

Possiting

Possiting is repeated regurgitation of small quantities of formula or breast milk soon after feeding. It is usually effortless and the amount of milk lost is not large. The infants are otherwise well but the effect of persistent dribbling onto clothes and bedclothes may be unpleasant.

Possiting is due to immaturity of the sphincter mechanism at the lower end of the oesophagus allowing liquid food to reflux up into the oesophagus, so called 'physiological' gastro-oesophageal reflux (GOR). Oesphagitis may occur with pathological GOR, or in babies who are very hungry feeders and swallow air which distends the stomach and reduces the competence of the sphincter.

Physiological GOR often improves following the introduction of solids and usually resolves by one year of age. However, in some children it persists well into the first year of life, but will eventually stop. The following criteria suggest pathological degrees of GOR requiring further investigation and treatment:

- inadequate weight gain
- feed refusal or pain on feeding
- blood in vomit
- recurrent cough, wheezing, or choking suggesting aspiration
- episodes of apnoea.

Whereas possiting is common, such complications are rare. Babies who show any of these features should be referred to a paediatrician for further assessment.

It is very tempting to blame possiting on the infant's feed and to use its presence as an excuse for switching from one formula to another. There is no evidence at all to justify this. The only relationship between possiting and food is the fact that by thickening the food the chance of possiting is reduced and this is a recognized method of management.

In cases where the possiting is frequent enough to be a real nuisance, a careful appraisal of feeding technique may be helpful, ensuring that the baby is not taking too much feed and does not take its feed too quickly thus swallowing air. Sitting the baby up for an hour after feeding will reduce the risk of regurgitation as an effect of gravity.

Feed thickeners

If these measures fail, thickening the bottle feed with an appropriate thickening agent may alleviate symptoms. Careful consideration should be given to the referral of such cases before further steps are taken.

There are several types of feed thickeners available (Table 7.1). In the majority of babies who possit, an instant thickener is most

Table 7.1. Feed thickeners

	Quantity required (per 100 ml feed)	Comments
Cornflower/ Arrowroot	2–4 g	4 kcal/g Requires cooking No prescription
Instant Carobel	0.3–1.5 g (Scoop provided)	Mainly non-digestible May cause bulky stool Requires prescription
Nestargel	0.5–1 g (Scoop provided)	Mainly non-digestible May cause bulky stools Requires prescription
Thixo-D	1–3 g (Scoop provided)	3.9 kcal/g Requires prescription
Vitaquick	1–3 g (Scoop provided)	4 kcal/g Requires prescription
Thick and easy	1–3 g	4 kcal/g Requires prescription

Note: Also available Enfamil AR—a complete pre-thickened infant formula.

appropriate and simple to use; some also provide energy which is beneficial in infants who also have poor weight gain. These thickeners can be added directly to the feed immediately prior to feeding. Cornflour can also be used as a thickener but requires cooking and must be prepared carefully following these instructions:

1. Mix powder to a paste with required volume of boiled water in clean, preferably sterile pan.
2. Bring the mixture to the boil, stirring continuously as though making custard.
3. Once it has thickened, the mixture can be poured into the feeding bottle.
4. Top up to required volume by adding boiled water.
5. Add required amount of infant formula powder.
6. Mix feed in usual way.

Note: The milk powder is added after cooking to prevent over-concentration and the destruction of heat-labile nutrients.

The feed thickener should be introduced initially at the lower concentration and the feed gradually thickened further if necessary. It is important to remember that all the feeding equipment and the utensils used in feed preparation should be sterilized in the normal way. The thickened feed may be too thick for the baby to suck through the usual teat and a larger hole teat or a special teat for thickened feeds should be used.

Infant Gaviscon and other anti-reflux antacid preparations should not be used to treat possiting. They contain sodium, which could lead to hypernatraemia and large amounts of aluminium, which is potentially toxic in young infants who are able to absorb aluminium from the gastrointestinal tract.

Feed thickeners can be offered to breast-fed babies as a thick paste on a spoon immediately before and after the feed.

In older babies (over three months) who possit, early weaning onto solids may be indicated. If possiting persists a combination of solids and thickened drinks may be useful. The feed thickeners mentioned above can also be used to thicken juices and water. It is above all essential to reassure the parents that in the absence of other symptoms this is not a serious condition and will eventually clear up even if they have to wait until the baby's first birthday.

More recently, prethickened infant formulae have become available. These are simple to mix as they are prepared like infant formula, however they do not allow for varying thickness and are therefore less flexible. There may be a danger of under- or over-concentration in order to achieve the required thickness. This in turn has the potential for under- or over-nutrition with its associated problems.

Vomiting

Persistent projectile vomiting developing around two weeks of age may indicate pyloric stenosis, particularly if associated with weight loss or cessation of weight gain. Community health workers should always seek help and advice in such cases. Bile stained vomiting should prompt immediate referral for a surgical opinion.

Almost all babies have the occasional unexplained vomit and the list of possible causes is extensive. Growth failure suggests that vomiting is significant.

Babies who are overfed may vomit because their gastric capacity is simply too small to cope with the volume of feed taken. Occasionally this increased volume will be an indirect consequence of over diluted formula, where the baby compensates for the low caloric density of the feed by taking a greater volume.

Food intolerance may cause vomiting but this is usually associated with diarrhoea and/or poor weight gain or other signs such as skin reactions. Food intolerance is discussed in Chapter 9.

A persistently vomiting baby is potentially seriously ill and requires careful assessment to identify the cause. It is dangerous to switch formulas in such babies on a speculative basis.

Rumination and habitual vomiting

Infants may learn how to regurgitate food from the stomach which they then chew and re-swallow. The techniques the infants use are either, to push the fingers into the mouth and so stimulate the gag reflex, or to use the tongue to produce the same effect. The baby may learn to ruminate only when not being watched. If the food losses are sufficient, failure to thrive may result. Babies likely to develop rumination are:

• infants with gastro-oesophageal reflux
• some developmentally delayed babies
• those who have been socially deprived and understimulated.

Management consists of:

• preventing fingers being pushed into the mouth
• thickening feeds
• early weaning
• distraction of the child after he has been fed
• increased personal attention.

Colic

Three-month or evening colic is a common functional condition of young babies which may be very distressing to the infant and cause considerable parental anxiety and stress, but which is ultimately self-limiting and harmless. Infants, usually between six weeks and three months of age, have repeated episodes, characteristically in the early evening. They cry, often yell, draw up their legs and show every evidence of spasmodic abdominal pain. The cause of colic is poorly understood, but pain may arise when muscle in the bowel wall goes into spasm. It varies a great deal in severity and duration. What causes this to happen is unknown but there have been attempts to incriminate feeding practices and foods given to babies with the inevitable tendency to manipulate the baby's diet to try to eliminate symptoms. Various studies have failed to show convincingly that there is a nutritional basis to the condition. The fact is that evening colic occurs in breast- and bottle-fed babies and infants fed either cows' milk or soya-based formulas. It has been suggested that cows' milk based feeds are more likely to be associated with colic than breast or soya formulas, yet babies changed to soya fail to show significant clinical improvement when account is taken of the natural tendency for symptoms to improve with time. It is claimed that breast-feeding mothers reduce colic in their babies if they limit their intake of cows' milk, but the evidence for this is tenuous. Certainly if mothers choose to reduce their own milk intake they should ensure that they have an adequate calcium intake. Very occasionally colic is related to cows' milk protein intolerance and a trial of a soya or hydrolysed formula is justified (see Chapter 9).

The medical profession has little to offer at present. Old-fashioned remedies such as alcohol-free gripe water, which contains peppermint extract and some other herbal constituents are worth trying. Some mothers have found fennel drinks to be useful and this appears to be perfectly safe; however, it is important to note that not all herbal remedies are safe and they should be used with caution. Sometimes, simply giving a drink of warm water can help. The most important role of health professionals is to give reassurance that the baby is not seriously ill and that the problem will eventually resolve. Parents who find the condition intolerable may often have other problems which are placing them under stress and attention should be given to proper support through health visitors and midwives. Above all the impression that the baby is abnormal in any way should be carefully avoided.

There is no justification for switching from one cows' milk based formula to another. Colic should not be used as a reason to stop breast-feeding.

Wind

Babies habitually swallow air while feeding. This is particularly likely to occur if the infant takes its feeds too fast, or conversely, if for any reason feeding is slowed down by faulty technique. The resulting excessively large gastric bubble causes distention of the stomach and distress. It can also result in excessive possiting. Some babies just seem to be more 'windy' than others. It is not serious but can lead to distress for both parents and baby. At present, the main danger is that wind will be blamed on the formula and ascribed to 'allergy'.

As with all digestive problems in the early weeks the principle of correct management is to establish that there is nothing seriously wrong with the baby, to reassure the mother, and to examine the feeding technique. A firm clear statement that the wind is most unlikely to be due to the nature of the milk may prevent unnecessary switching of feeds or abandonment of breast-feeding.

The teat should be checked to make sure the hole is neither too large nor too small. The method used for mixing the feed should also be checked to make sure it does not include vigorous shaking of the bottle immediately prior to feeding; this traps air bubbles and may exacerbate the problem. The mother should be watched feeding the baby and advised on how to prevent air swallowing, how to slow down the rate of feeding, and how to 'wind' the baby, frequently, if air swallowing is a major problem. Some of the more common mistakes in feeding which contribute to wind include not tilting the bottle correctly, thus allowing the teat to become empty, and not removing the bottle from the baby's mouth at intervals to prevent the teat collapsing. This again encourages the baby to gulp air. Fig. 7.2 illustrates the correct position for bottle-feeding. If it is difficult to remove the teat from the baby's mouth during feeding the use of a bottle with a disposable bag interior may be helpful as this collapses as the baby feeds. There is also some evidence to suggest that the new tilted feeding bottles can be helpful in reducing wind.

With the breast-fed infant it is also important to check the feeding position ensuring that the baby has a good seal around the nipple.

Constipation

Constipation (the difficult passage of hard stools) is a common complaint during infancy. Breast-fed babies are rarely

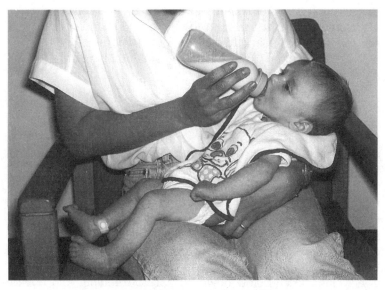

Fig. 7.2. Correct bottle-feeding position.

constipated, probably due to the more complete absorption of fats in breast milk leaving low levels of calcium soaps, which are stool hardeners. Additionally, the acid, fermentative stools of the breast-fed baby are softer and more bulky than those of the formula-fed baby. It is not unusual for breast-fed babies to pass many soft stools daily which the unwary might mistake for diarrhoea, although some infants seem to store it all up for an occasional massive, explosive episode.

Parents may become disproportionately anxious about their babies' bowel habits and often it is reassurance that is required, rather than action because the infants are not truly constipated. Artificially-fed babies who have at least one stool every other day without excessive straining are unlikely to have serious problems.

Constipation is more common in formula-fed babies but in the absence of organic disease is rarely severe. Stools may be small, greenish, pellet-like, and occasionally these may be blood-streaked if a fissure develops. Fissures are painful and may perpetuate the constipation.

If constipation is a problem in young babies the following steps should be taken:

• check fluid intake is adequate
• ensure formula is being diluted correctly
• give drinks of boiled water or diluted fresh orange juice between feeds
• add 1 teaspoon of sugar to the bottle, this will give a higher osmolar feed which will draw fluid into the bowel and create a softer stool; use only as a short-term measure as it increases the calorie density of the feed.

If a baby is genuinely constipated, the introduction of solids at three months can help. Puréed fruits, vegetables, and cereals should be encouraged. Wholegrain cereals can be introduced gradually from six months of age and beans and pulses at a later stage. Pure bran is not recommended in young children and is not necessary if the fibre content of the diet is gradually increased using food naturally high in fibre. It is important to ensure that the infant has a good fluid intake as fibre absorbs water.

Severe constipation from the time of birth should be investigated and raises the possibility of Hirschsprung's disease or anatomical abnormality. Constipation in the older child is discussed in Chapter 3.

Choking episodes

One of the most frightening things that can happen to a parent is to see their young child choke on food. It can happen with liquids or solids, but is particularly likely at the time when the infant is beginning to take solids and may have to deal with a lump which causes him to gag. Some specific foods are more likely to present a choking hazard in young children and they should be avoided unless presented in a ground or puréed form; they include:

• peanuts
• raisins
• grapes
• raw vegetables
• boiled sweets.

The reader should note that nuts in any form may not be suitable for children under one year of age, especially where there is a family history of food allergy (see Chapter 9). Other foods may also cause choking, especially if the child stuffs too much in his mouth or is running whilst eating. Choking can be avoided if the child is offered suitable foods and eats sitting in a high chair or at the table, allowing him to concentrate on chewing and swallowing.

The occasional child seems to have special difficulty with, or an aversion to, lumpy food and full evaluation by a speech therapist and/or clinical psychologist skilled in the use of desensitization techniques may be helpful.

There are some important organic disorders which may be associated with choking. Repeated episodes should be treated seriously and warrant referral for further investigation.

Overfeeding and underfeeding

Most babies appear to have an internal caloric sensor which enables them to control the amount of energy they take in. Although it is the size of the baby which will determine the average intake, there is much variation in the quantity of food babies require to achieve a normal growth rate. The reasons for this are still not fully understood but there is evidence that underlying rates of metabolism vary. Thus, some babies will require as little as 140 ml of formula per kilo per day, while others will require as much as 200 ml. Much so-called overfeeding or underfeeding is the result of too rigid application of norms. If a baby is well and growing at a normal rate, too much should not be made of the actual volume of intake. Concern may arise if a baby is obviously fat. Whether infants should be dieted is a controversial matter discussed in detail in Chapter 10.

Underfeeding should only be considered if a baby is failing to grow appropriately. Most infants will quickly signal their dissatisfaction if they are not getting enough. One exception to this principle is the problem of the underfed breast-fed baby and problems may arise if the baby is not fed sufficiently frequently. Very young infants may not cope with the consequently larger volumes per feed. While babies should be demand fed there are limits to the size of the gap between feeds which are acceptable.

Parents are often anxious about the exact volume of feed their babies should take. Table 2.9 is an attempt to offer an approximate guide to such questions, but it is very important that a flexible attitude be taken to this matter. Rigid adherence to predetermined figures would lead to inappropriate feeding of most babies. More important is the length of time an infant should be allowed to go without a feed. While it is highly unlikely that a normal baby would come to significant harm, fasts of longer than 8 hours under the age of three months are undesirable.

Errors in bottle-feeding technique

Faulty technique in artificially-fed babies is a common cause of problems. These are mainly simple mechanical errors.

Size of teat hole

The size of the teat hole can be important. There are old stories about babies being fed with teats with no hole at all and clearly this would have unfortunate consequences! If the hole is too small, feeding will become a struggle with frustration of both baby and mother. If it is too big, the baby may take its feed too quickly, distending the stomach, causing 'wind', and possibly aggravating colic symptoms. A good test to check the size of the teat hole is to turn the bottle upside down and allow milk to drip out. The ideal size of teat hole for most babies allows droplets to come out so close together that they almost form a constant stream.

Bottle propping

Putting a bottle into the mouth of a reclining baby and letting it 'get on with it' is a practice which should be deplored. There is a real risk of aspiration and it is not safe for a young baby to be left sucking on a bottle unsupervised. Bottle propping may also deprive the child of important socialization and interaction and will contribute to the risk of dental caries in a child with teeth.

Babies who are difficult to feed

There is group of babies who appear to have been appropriately managed who nevertheless prove difficult to feed and such infants should always be referred to a paediatrician for assessment. They may be suffering from a range of organic disorders, including potentially treatable metabolic defects, or may be showing the early signs of neurological dysfunction such as cerebral palsy. Finally, there are some babies, otherwise normal, who appear to have a functional problem with sucking and swallowing which may require the special skills of the speech therapist to overcome (Fig. 7.3).

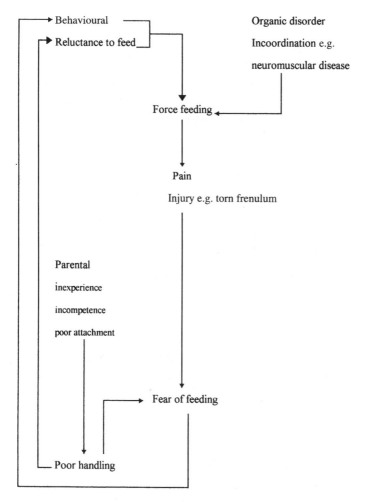

Fig. 7.3. Feeding difficulty in infancy.

Similar feeding difficulties can occur because of parental inadequacies, but by the time the baby comes to medical attention it may be impossible to resolve how the problem began. A careful psychosocial assessment of the family is therefore essential.

Whatever the origins, the baby will usually present as a fractious infant who tends to stiffen and curl up or arch his back when attempts are made at feeding. The baby will either resist the teat being placed in the mouth or simply refuse to suck. If the baby can be induced to feed he may appear to have difficulties with sucking or swallowing, cough, splutter, and choke. The time taken to get the infant to consume an appropriate volume of feed may be impracticably long, so that virtually the whole day is taken up with the struggle from one bottle to the next. Little wonder that parents become exhausted and are driven to the end of their tether. Very occasionally a child will seem indifferent to feeding from birth. It is possible that such infants have a primary disorder of appetite.

Successful management requires reassurance to the parents and understanding of their difficulties, together with an explanation that this is a common experience and will resolve.

It may be appropriate to recommend an alternative teat for the bottle-fed baby who is having difficulty sucking. Sometimes a small soft preterm teat can be helpful, as it may be easier for the baby to feed with this. For the baby who is having difficulties with solids, a change in the type of spoon or in the texture of the solid foods may help. The positioning of the baby during feeding can make it difficult for him to swallow or may aggravate any stiffening or arching. Experimenting with different feeding positions can alleviate this but should be done under professional supervision.

Irrespective of the underlying cause, the baby may eventually present a feeding problem to everyone, including experienced professionals, particularly if the parents have reached the force-feeding stage. Psychology and speech therapy colleagues can provide invaluable advice regarding feeding strategies and behavioural interventions. Home visits by speech therapists and outreach nurses give an opportunity to watch the mother feeding the baby so that feeding mechanisms can be assessed and technical deficiencies can be corrected. Input from the dietitian can help allay fears of nutritional inadequacies and prevent nutritional deficiencies. Continued support from the health visitor and outreach nurses may be required over months or years.

Force-feeding

Force-feeding is the end-result of several different processes. It is important because of the direct dangers it holds for the baby and because of what it tells us of the mother–child relationship. Its primary cause is the sense in the feeder that the baby is not feeding properly.

This perception may be mistaken and reflect the unrealistic expectations of a young, inexperienced mother. Alternatively, if a good attachment has not formed between mother and baby, tolerance of the infant may be low and any slight 'misdemeanour' by the baby provokes irritation. The tolerance level may also be reduced if the mother is depressed or unhappy. Sometimes the source of the trouble is not the mother but the fact that many people are feeding the baby, who is sensitive to an atmosphere of inconsistency or disorder.

Whatever starts off the process, the effect is similar. The feeder will exert pressure on the bottle forcing the teat into the baby's mouth. This will induce discomfort and eventually panic so that the reluctant or incompetent baby becomes more difficult to feed and parental frustration and forceful feeding becomes progressively more intense.

The process of force-feeding will have a number of untoward effects. It will cause the baby to fear feeding because of the discomfort it engenders. The infant may begin to scream at the first sight of the bottle or introduction of the teat. Feeding times will become a real ordeal and effective feeding may become impossible culminating in failure to thrive. A depressed or unhappy mother will feel increasingly incapable and guilty, thus accentuating the emotional upset.

Force-feeding is an important harbinger of non-accidental injury. The frenulum of the tongue or upper lip may be torn and injuries also occur to the palate and fauces. This will lead to extreme pain and screaming and may culminate with more serious non-accidental injury, particularly facial bruising, rib fractures, and shaking injuries. A tell-tale sign is a semi-circle of fingertip bruises round the mouth and chin. It is remarkable how common the association is between such external injuries and evidence of force-feeding. If the injuries have been caused by someone other than the mother she may find the whole matter inexplicable but it has to be recognized that force-feeding may be part of a much more serious pattern of abuse and neglect outside the scope of this volume.

Management is similar to that of any baby who is difficult to feed but there should be no hesitation in admitting the baby, who may be at considerable risk, to hospital.

The dissatisfied baby

One of the commonest complaints encountered in the early weeks of life is that the baby is dissatisfied with the amount of feed being offered. This is often expressed by the statement that the mother cannot 'fill' the baby. In fact what is being described is really a baby who for some reason either does not settle after a feed or has frequent periods of crying or periods of crying which the mother perceives as excessive. This is less likely to be a problem with breast-fed babies and tends to be correlated with adverse home circumstances. Before ascribing these complaints to the baby's feeds, careful assessment of other possible causes should always be made.

Some babies require more food than others. Problems may arise if babies are fed to rigid schedules and parents advised to give fixed quantities of formula. Ideally all babies, should be fed on demand and given as much food as they will take. Because of the internal calorie sensor mechanism, as long as the feed is correctly prepared there will be no danger of excessive weight gain. Babies should never be hungry after a feed.

Parents who perceive that their baby is 'not satisfied' may do one of two things. They may either start the baby on solid foods or switch the formula, either on their own initiative or on the advice of family or health worker. Some writers argue that there is no harm in this and that realism dictates that these are practices which should simply be accommodated. While the case for some degree of flexibility is desirable, it seems very defeatist to accept practices which official recommendations continue to regard as undesirable. As we have already discussed in Chapter 2, the introduction of solids is based on the developmental readiness of the infant and not simply the chronological age (Table 7.2). There is potential harm to both early introduction of solids and formula switching and in accepting a false explanation for a phenomenon.

Early introduction of solids

During the 1960s it was widely accepted practice to introduce solids at a very early age. Several studies showed that most babies were on solids by six weeks of age and in some cases solids were being introduced during the first weeks of life. This was the era of excessive weight gain in early life and hypertonic dehydration. This was in part due to the use of formulas based on whole cows' milk and incorrect preparation, but there is evidence that solids given early formed part of the problem by increasing the caloric density of the feed. Early weaning may also increase the risk of coeliac disease possibly by exposing the baby to gluten during a most vulnerable period.

During the first weeks of life, perhaps because of the lack of secretory IgA, babies may be more vulnerable to sensitization by food allergens and it seems sensible to limit the range of such potential allergens to a minimum.

Adding solids to bottle

In the recent past, adding solids, particularly baby cereal to formula had become a widespread practice. Just why some parents do this is not clear but it may be conceived as a simpler way of feeding the baby or it may have been thought to help the baby sleep through the night. For whatever reason, this is an undesirable practice as it increases both the caloric density of the formula and the solute load. It may also encourage early weaning which for reasons already stated is considered undesirable.

Another, more subtle objection stems from the fact that feeding babies solids with a spoon during early weaning represents an important period of child–parent interaction which may have a bearing on intellectual and emotional development.

Table 7.2. Guidelines for progression of solid foods

Age in months	Feeding skills	Oral motor skills	Types of food	Suggested activities
0–4		Rooting reflex Sucking reflex Swallowing reflex Extrusion reflex	Breast milk Infant formula	Breast-feed or bottle-feed
5	Able to grasp objects voluntarily Learning to reach mouth with hands	Disappearance of extrusion reflex		Possible introduction of thinned cereal
6	Sits with balance while using hands	Transfers food from front of tongue to back	Infant cereal Strained fruit Strained vegetables	Prepare cereal with formula or breast milk to a semiliquid texture Use spoon Feed from a dish Advance to 1/3–1/2 cup cereal before adding fruits or vegetables

Table 7.2. (continued)

7	Improved grasp Mashes food with lateral movements of jaw Learns side-to-side or 'rotary' chewing	Infant cereal Strained to junior texture of fruits, vegetables, and meats	Thicken cereal to lumpier texture Sit in highchair with feet supported Introduce cup
8–10	Holds bottle without help Drinks from cup without spilling Decreases fluid intake and increases solids Coordinates hand-to-mouth movement	Juices Soft, mashed, or minced table foods	Begin finger foods Do not add salt, sugar, or fats to food Present soft foods in chunks ready for finger feeding

Table 7.2. (continued)

Age in months	Feeding skills	Oral motor skills	Types of food	Suggested activities
10–12	Feeds self	Tooth eruption	Soft, chopped table foods	Provide meals in pattern similar to rest of family
	Holds cup without help	Improved ability to bite and chew		Use cup at meals

Note: Reproduced with permission from: Queen, P.M. and Lang, C.E. (1993). *Handbook of pediatric nutrition.* Aspen Publishers Inc. Maryland, USA.

Switching feeds

Various studies have shown that for about 20–25% of babies the type of formula is changed during the first six weeks of life. This happens for a variety of reasons, the usual reason being that the baby was not satisfied or was allergic to the cows' milk preparation. Switching of feeds in Britain tends to be from one cows' milk formula to another, while in the United States the change is usually from cows' milk formula to soya. This latter tendency is seen increasingly in parts of Britain as well.

Most babies are started on whey-based feeds (see Chapter 2). This is because maternity services generally advocate them as they are most similar to breast milk. There is no theoretical reason why the formula should be changed to any other cows' milk based feed. Despite this, the rate of switching is high. Since babies are usually on a whey-based feed, the likelihood is that they will be switched to a casein-based feed, something which is reinforced by the mistaken belief that babies are less satisfied by whey than casein-based formulas. Some health professionals actually advocate that babies should be changed to casein-based feeds at three months. There is no evidence to suggest that this is necessary.

Is formula switching important? It can be argued that as a matter of consumer choice, there is no reason why parents should not shop around among a series of formulas, all approved for use as infant feed until they find the one they perceive as satisfactory. This 'free-market' view is open to some criticisms. First there is the philosophical issue that encouragement should not be given to ascribing cause incorrectly. If the baby's symptoms are not due to the nature of the feed it is inherently undesirable to suggest the opposite. The practical aspects of this principle are seen when delay occurs in the diagnosis of genuine disease because the parents abetted by health workers have indulged in a futile bout of formula swapping.

Further reading

Farber, S.D., Van Fossen, R.L., and Koontz, S.W. (1995). Quantitive and qualitive video analysis of infants feeding: Angled and straight-bottle feeding systems. *Journal of Pedatrics*, **126**, (6), S118–24.

Quinlan, P.T., Lockton, S., Irwin, J., and Lucas, A.L. (1995). The relationship between stool hardness and stool composition in breast- and formula-fed infants. *Journal of Pediatric Gastroenterology and Nutrition*, **20**, 81–90.

Taitz, L.S. and Scholey, E. (1989). Are babies more satisfied by casein based formulas? *Archives of Disease in Childhood*, **64**, 619–21.

8

....

Diarrhoea

Diarrhoea in infants and young children is defined as the frequent passage of watery stools. Excessive loss of intestinal contents, either acute or chronic, may have nutritional consequences through interruption of normal food intake, or as a result of maldigestion and malabsorption of nutrients.

Acute diarrhoea

During short lived episodes of acute onset diarrhoea the main risk to the child is dehydration and associated electrolyte disturbance. With more than a billion diarrhoeal episodes amongst children each year world-wide, diarrhoea is second only to malnutrition as a cause of infant death. It is also a major factor in pushing children with borderline nutrition into full-blown protein-calorie malnutrition.

In developed countries, particularly with improvements in infant feeding it has become a much less severe condition than in the past, yet in the UK still remains one of the commonest reasons for admission to hospital for children under five. Younger infants are at greatest risk of dehydration since they have higher basal fluid requirements and immature renal compensatory mechanisms. They are also more likely to develop complications secondary to damage of the gastrointestinal mucosa, such as lactose, cows' milk, and soya protein intolerance.

Breast milk provides protection against gastro-enteritis not only because it is free of pathogens which cause diarrhoeal disease but also because it contains anti-infective agents such as secretory IgA and lactoferrin. Bottle feeds and solid food can be contaminated with bacteria particularly where there is lack of refrigeration, poor hygeine, and contaminated water supplies.

Causes

Most acute sickness and diarrhoea (gastro-enteritis) is infectious in origin. The causative organisms are most commonly viral (rotavirus), but may be bacterial (e.g. salmonella, shigella, campylobacter, E. coli) or protozoal (*giardia lamblia*). Rotavirus and enterotoxogenic bacteria are the most important causes of acute diarrhoea in young children. In the UK, around half of children admitted to hospital with acute gastro-enteritis have no organism isolated from the stools.

A number of different mechanisms contribute to infectious diarrhoea including:

- disruption of normal cell transport processes in the gastrointestinal mucosa
- an osmotic load from non-absorbed solutes in the intestine
- deranged intestinal permeability
- disruption of normal bowel motility.

Nutritional effects

Acute diarrhoea in otherwise healthy children generally does not affect nutrition but in malnourished children it can lead to a further deterioration of nutritional status. Food intolerance, either primary, or as a secondary complication of gastro-enteritis is an important cause of persistent diarrhoea and is discussed in Chapter 9. Malnutrition, compounded by specific deficiencies such as zinc, adversely affects immunity and predisposes to further infection, leading in time to impairment of pancreatic and gastric function. A vicious cycle is thereby set up where repeated infections predispose to worsening malnutrition and further infection.

Management

Managing the child with acute diarrhoea involves prevention and treatment of dehydration with its associated electrolyte disturbance, together with maintenance or resumption of adequate nutrition.

Dehydration as a consequence of diarrhoea is often categorized as mild, moderate, or severe based on the percentage loss of body weight. Mild dehydration corresponds to a loss of less than 5%, moderate dehydration to 5–10% loss, and severe dehydration when more than 10% of body weight has been lost. However, accurate clinical assessment of dehydration is difficult (Table 8.1) and the severity tends to be overestimated; in hospital, this results in unnecessary use of intravenous rehydration. If a recent weight is available, comparison with current weight gives the best measure of fluid deficit. In general, only a very small proportion of children admitted to hospital in the UK with acute diarrhoea are found to be moderately or severely dehydrated. An outline of management is given in Table 8.2.

The majority of children can usually be managed quite safely at home. A glucose and electrolyte preparation (oral rehydration solution, ORS) should be given and the desired fluid intake and feed schedule written down for parents. Small amounts of fluid

Table 8.1. Features of dehydration

2–3%	Thirst, mild reduction in urine output
5%	Thirst, reduction in urine; slightly sunken eyes and fontanelle; alteration in skin tone
6–9%	Sunken eyes with loss of eyeball tension; sunken fontanelle, loss of skin turgor; marked thirst and decrease in urine output; increasing apathy
10% +	All the above, plus poor perfusion, rapid heart rate, weak pulse, low blood pressure

Table 8.2. Management of acute gastro-enteritis

Dehydration absent or mild:
- the aim is to prevent dehydration
- provide clear instructions to parents
- careful observation during illness to check for signs of dehydration
- if there is vomiting, small volumes of fluid may need to be given frequently (for example using a teaspoon)

Infants

Breast-fed:	- continue breast-feeds
	- if ORS tolerated, reintroduce solids after 4 hours when rehydrated
	- offer supplements of ORS for duration of diarrhoeal episode
Formula-fed:	- stop milk feeds; stop solids
	- give 25 ml/kg ORS + any estimated fluid deficit over 4 hours
	- if ORS tolerated, reintroduce normal full strength formula
	- if formula tolerated, reintroduce solids
	- continue to offer ORS supplements for the duration of the diarrhoeal episode

Children
- give ORS in a volume equal to maintenance requirements + any estimated fluid deficit over 4 hours
- if tolerated, reintroduce normal diet
- continue to offer ORS supplements for duration of diarrhoeal episode

>5% Dehydration present or uncontrolled vomiting:
- intravenous fluids required
    - admit to hospital for intravenous fluids
    - recommence normal diet after 24 hours

---

given frequently are often tolerated even when vomiting has been a prominent symptom. The various preparations available in the UK and which are suitable for home therapy are listed in Table 8.3. Solutions containing higher concentrations of sodium (e.g. WHO solution—90 mmol/l) are not widely used in Europe

Table 8.3. Some oral rehydration preparations

Product (oral powder)	Glucose (mmol)	Sodium (mmol)	Potassium (mmol)	Chloride (mmol)
Diocalm Junior	111	60	20	50
Dioralyte	90	60	20	60
(effervescent tablets)	(90)	(60)	(25)	(45)
Electrolade	111	50	20	40
Gluco-lyte	200	35	20	37
Rapolyte	111	60	20	50
Rehydrat	91*	50	20	50

Note: All concentrations are given for the product diluted to 1000 ml according to manu-facturers instructions.
When preparing these products for infants all water should be freshly boiled and cooled.
*Also contains 94 mmol sucrose and 1–2 mmol fructose.

where viral gastro-enteritis is most common and stool sodium losses are lower than they would be in countries where cholera is prevalent. Home-made recipes combining 'a pinch of salt and a teaspoon of sugar' are notoriously inaccurate and should not be used. Carbonated drinks which have been allowed to go 'flat' should also be discouraged as a form of treatment since they contain inappropriate electrolytes and a high osmolar load which may make diarrhoea worse. In general, anti-diarrhoeal drugs and antibiotics are contra-indicated, although still widely misused.

Feeding with solids

Once dehydration has been corrected it is unnecessary to starve the child of enteral nutrition. Unfortunately, it is still common for a period of starvation ('resting the bowel') or slow building up over several days of dilute milk feeds ('regrading') to be recommended, despite the fact that there is no scientific basis for this approach. Breast-feeding should continue during the episode of diarrhoea. Caution is often recommended when reintroducing formula milk to infants under six months of age, and there is still no general agreement on how (full strength or dilute) and when to introduce feeds. A recent European study has shown that complete resumption of normal feeding (including lactose containing formula) after only 4 hours of rehydration with oral rehydration solution did not lead to worsening of diarrhoea, increased duration of diarrhoea, increased vomiting, or lactose intolerance, but did result in significant weight gain compared to the late feeding group, where normal food was introduced after 24 hours. The 'Working Group on Early Feeding in Acute Gastroenteritis' of the European Society of Paediatric Gastroenterology and Nutrition (ESPGAN) now consider that in mild and moderate dehydration there should be a 3 to 4 hour period of rehydration with ORS, followed by reintroduction of normal feeding. Supplementation with ORS to compensate for continuing fluid and electrolyte losses in the stool should be given for the duration of the diarrhoeal illness.

Admission to hospital

Although most diarrhoeal disease is mild and can be treated effectively at home, the following constitute indications for admission:

- clinical signs of dehydration
- vomiting of glucose and electrolyte solution, or inability to comply with oral rehydration advice for whatever reason
- persistence or recurrence of diarrhoea
- suspected surgical conditions (e.g. intussusception, appendicitis)
- poor social circumstances/lack of supervision
- short history of profuse diarrhoea
- pre-existing medical condition which may worsen with diarrhoea (e.g. diabetes mellitus).

There should be a lower threshold for admitting young infants under six months of age because of the relatively greater risk of dehydration. Many children from poor socio-economic backgrounds are admitted to hospital and have not been seen by a general practitioner. This emphasizes the need for a better community-based infrastructure so that such children can be managed at home. Although children with moderate–severe dehydration admitted to hospital in countries like the UK will be given intravenous fluids, in countries where this therapy is not available, ORS is successfully employed.

Continuing diarrhoea and the use of special formulas

Continuing diarrhoea may indicate:

• lactose intolerance
• milk protein intolerance.

The former diagnosis can be confirmed by testing watery stool for reducing substances. On the hospital ward this is simply done by mixing five drops of stool fluid with ten drops of water and adding one Clinitest (Ames) tablet. A colour change in the specimen can be compared with a chart which indicates whether reducing substances are present. The diagnosis of lactose intolerance is usually based on the finding of 1% or more of reducing substances in the stool. The presence of lactose in the stool can be confirmed by sugar chromatography in the laboratory.

In the first instance, this can be managed by a return to glucose and electrolyte solution for 24 hours, and then a build up to full strength milk over several days. If lactose intolerance persists, a trial of lactose-free soya-based infant formula is warranted. Alternatively, a hydrolysed whey- or casein-based formula may be used (see Table 9.1), which some consider to be the preferred option. It is usually possible to reintroduce ordinary feeds within a week or two once weight loss has been regained.

When recurrent diarrhoea occurs after reintroduction of milk, but without lactose in the stool, the possibility of secondary cows' milk protein intolerance must be considered. An extensively hydrolysed protein formula should be given for a few weeks with cautious reintroduction of a milk-based feed. Occasionally hydrolysed feeds are not tolerated and then an amino acid based feed (Neocate, Scientific Hospital Supplies) will be necessary. The use of these highly specialized formulas requires careful nutritional assessment and management and should be done under the joint supervision of a paediatrician and paediatric dietitian.

Chronic diarrhoea

There is a long list of causes of intractable diarrhoea associated with failure to thrive during infancy which require highly specialized investigation and management. Age of onset can be a clue to the aetiology, but in some children a cause cannot be found. Some of these important diagnoses are discussed elsewhere (see Chapters 9 and 12), and include:

• post-gastro-enteritis syndrome (persistent diarrhoea after an acute infectious gastro-enteritis)
• coeliac disease
• immunodeficiency
• autoimmune enteropathy.

'Diarrhoea de retour'

Many parents who have recently migrated to Europe like to take their young children back to their homelands to meet their relatives. The change in bacterial flora and food often causes diarrhoea which in severe cases may go on to cause malnutrition and intractable diarrhoea on return to Britain. A similar condition was first described in France in children returning there from Algeria and Morocco. It is important to recognize this entity early and not to attempt domiciliary treatment with starvation and re-grading as this will aggravate the situation. These children will often have developed secondary lactose, cow's milk, or soya intolerance, and the problem may be complicated by worm infestation or infection with unusual bacterial organisms. The introduction of oral feeding can be very difficult; a period of parenteral nutrition and use of an elemental or modular feed using comminuted chicken (Chix, Cow and Gate) as the nitrogen source may be required. Full recovery sometimes takes many months.

All babies with protracted diarrhoea require thorough investigation in a paediatric gastro-enterology unit. It is hazardous to assume diagnoses such as lactose or milk protein intolerance without careful assessment.

Further reading

Brown, K.H., Peerson, J.M., and Fontaine, O. (1994). Use of nonhuman milks in the dietary management of young children with acute diarrhoea: a meta-analysis of clinical trials. *Pediatrics*, **93**, 17–27.

Conway, S.P., Phillips, R.R., and Panday, S. (1990). Admission to hospital with gastroenteritis. *Archives of Disease in Childhood*, **65**, 579–84.

Goodburn, S., Mattosinho, S., Mongi, P., and Waterston, T. (1991). Management of childhood diarrhoea by pharmacists and parents: is Britain lagging behind the Third World? *British Medical Journal*, **302**, 440–3.

Walker-Smith, J.A. (1992). Advances in the management of gastroenteritis in children. *British Journal of Hospital Medicine*, **48**, 582–5.

9

Food allergy and intolerance

Adverse reactions to ingested food cause a wide variety of symptoms and diseases for which the general descriptive terms sensitivity and intolerance are useful. These terms can be applied to a reaction with an unknown mechanism as well as to a clearly defined metabolic, pharmacologic, or immuno-pathologic process. The following definitions have been suggested:

Food intolerance or sensitivity: a reproducible, unpleasant reaction, not psychologically based, to a specific food or ingredient. Mechanisms include enzyme deficiency (e.g. lactase deficiency), pharmacologic effects (e.g. those caused by caffeine), non-immunologic histamine-releasing effects (e.g. those caused by certain shellfish), and direct irritation (e.g. by gastric acid in oesophagitis, colonic flatus in carbohydrate intolerance).

Food allergy or food hypersensitivity: a form of food intolerance in which there are both reproducible food intolerance and evidence of an abnormal immunologic reaction to food (mediated by antibody or T lymphocytes, or both).

Psychologically based food reactions (food aversions): this may be when the subject avoids food for psychological reasons, or when there is an unpleasant bodily reaction caused by emotions associated with the food (rather than by the food itself) and does not occur when the food is given in an unrecognizable form.

Food intolerance

Food 'intolerance' is the preferred term when referring to adverse reactions to food as it does not imply any particular mechanism, whereas 'allergy' implies an underlying immunological mechanism, which may be food specific antibodies, immune complexes, or cell mediated reactions. Cow's milk, eggs, nuts, and fruit are the most commonly implicated foods in childhood, and food intolerance appears to be more common during infancy than in adult life. In a North American study 16% of children were said to have had reactions to fruit or fruit juice and 28% to other food by the age of three. One problem with defining the frequency of food intolerance is that parents' reports often prove unreliable when compared with double-blind challenges.

There is a recognized association between food intolerance and atopic eczema. Atopic individuals are at risk of developing eczema, hay fever, acute allergic (type 1, IgE mediated) reactions and asthma. As many as 30% of the population are atopic so that allergic conditions, usually mild and often transitory, are common. If both parents are affected then it is highly likely that their children will also develop allergy in one form or the other.

Many, but not all, atopic people have elevated levels of the immunoglobulin IgE in their blood. Not all allergic children have food allergy. Inhaled allergens, pollen, animal dander, and the excreta of house dust mites are actually much more important allergens causing hay fever, allergic rhinitis and conjunctivitis, and most significantly, asthma. Just why children with the same underlying tendency have such varying reactions remains a mystery but nevertheless a child with one type of allergy is more likely to have or develop another type. For example babies with eczema are more likely to develop asthma later in life even if the eczema clears up.

The neonatal gastrointestinal tract is permeable to the passage of milk proteins and small water soluble molecules, particularly in the preterm infant. The biological and clinical significance of this observation remains unclear. Secretory IgA, with its capacity to agglutinate intra luminal antigens, is the first line of immunologic defence at the mucosal surface. High titres of IgA in colostrum help to protect the mucosal surfaces of the breast-fed newborn infants, while circulating immunoglobulins (IgG and IgM) represent a further line of defence against absorbed antigens. In babies in general, and those from allergic families in particular, it may well be prudent to:

- exclusively breast-feed for the first 4–6 months of life
- avoid early introduction of foods which have a high potential for sensitization (e.g. egg, wheat, nuts).

It is well known that infants can be sensitized by allergens appearing in the mother's milk, and that some babies already have specific IgE antibodies to cows' milk protein at birth suggesting that prenatal sensitization can occur.

Acute reactions

Many individuals will have had at least one episode in which apparently out of the blue they develop severe abdominal cramp with or without vomiting and diarrhoea associated with a generalized itchy rash with wheals and urticaria, swelling of the eyes or lips, and malaise which disappears as fast as it appears. Such reactions are almost certainly due to some component of food, often unidentifiable. Similar symptoms are frequently triggered by drug treatment. IgE is the immunoglobulin involved and histamine among the substances released which produce the reaction. Occasionally it becomes obvious that a particular food is the offending agent because similar reactions occur whenever that food is eaten.

At the less severe end of the spectrum is the condition of recurrent urticaria (hives) which is a nuisance and not dangerous and may be a specific response to an easily identifiable food such as strawberries.

Acute reactions do occur during infancy and are most likely to be due to cows' milk or egg protein sensitivity. Obvious swelling, redness, or even blistering of the lips or skin round the mouth occurs on contact followed by vomiting and diarrhoea. In the experience of the authors, egg is the most likely cause of this type of reaction but similar reactions may occur with cow's milk, peanut- or wheat-containing foods.

At the extreme end of severity is the anaphylactic reaction with sudden onset of bronchospasm and circulatory failure. Some individuals develop swelling in the mouth immediately on contact with the food, which may progress to laryngeal oedema and respiratory obstruction causing severe breathing difficulty. Sensitivity to nuts can be one cause of this extreme response. Peanut allergy appears to be both a lifelong problem and increasing in prevalence. In addition to avoiding the obvious sources of peanuts, careful scrutiny of manufactured and baked products is required as many contain peanut derivatives and are not labelled as such. Products containing peanut oil may contain traces of peanut protein, and must therefore be avoided. Those affected may need to carry a syringe of adrenaline ('Epipen') for emergency intramuscular injection.

When acute reactions occur with specific foods avoidance of that food is the obvious solution but the lengths to which one would go must depend on the severity of the symptoms. An individual who gets a few hives from strawberries who has passion for the fruit might well decide the transient discomfort is a small price to pay for the delight. On the other hand an individual who develops severe laryngeal oedema at the merest contact with Brazil nut would have to avoid them at all costs.

Delayed reactions

Reactions to foods are often delayed hours, or even days after ingestion and a number of different immunological mechanisms (e.g. cell mediated; immune complex formation) are implicated. One example is cow's milk protein intolerance (CMPI) which affects around 2.5% of infants.

Cow's milk protein intolerance

CMPI is the clinical syndrome or syndromes resulting from sensitization of an individual child to one or more proteins in cow's milk. This may be a primary problem in which there appear to be no predisposing factors, or secondary to acute gastro-enteritis. Permeability of small bowel mucosa to antigen and the control of the antigen and the immune response to it once absorbed may both be important in the pathogenesis. Primary CMPI is possibly due to a disturbance in the local immune system for antigen control, particularly antigen exclusion. The secondary syndrome can result when gut damage secondary to infection makes the mucosa abnormally permeable to antigen entry. An immunodeficiency state, such as transient IgA deficiency, may be an important predisposing factor for both syndromes.

In most children gastrointestinal symptoms (vomiting, diarrhoea, colic, failure to thrive) develop within the first six months of life. There may be a family history of atopy, except in cases secondary to gastro-enteritis. Symptoms can come on acutely, mimicking acute infectious gastro-enteritis, or may develop more insidiously. In the breast-fed infant, the disease may present following introduction of infant formula, and very occasionally an anaphylactic reaction is observed. Cow's milk proteins can be detected in breast milk in many mothers and some studies have shown that about 0.5% of exclusively breast-fed infants develop CMPI. Other presentations of CMPI include:

- respiratory: wheeze, rhinitis, asthma
- dermatological: atopic dermatitis, urticaria, laryngeal oedema
- behavioural: irritability, crying, milk refusal.

Of those infants with predominantly gastrointestinal symptoms some present only with colic or constipation, whilst others are well except for blood in the stools. These have an underlying colitis and histological examination of colonic mucosa characteristically shows infiltration by eosinophils.

Diagnosis of CMPI is based largely on clinical history and the following criteria are widely used:

- definite disappearance of symptoms after each of two dietary eliminations of cow's milk and cow's milk products
- recurrence of identical symptoms after one challenge, and
- exclusion of lactose intolerance and coincidental infection.

In children with chronic diarrhoeal symptoms jejunal biopsy is sometimes performed. Histological examination of the jejunum reveals patchy abnormalities with partial atrophy of the villi. The removal of cow's milk protein from the diet will lead to immediate and dramatic clinical improvement. There has been some controversy as to whether these ill babies should be fed soya formula or one of the hydrolysed protein formulas (Table 9.1). We recommend the latter despite the greater cost, as there is a significant risk of development of soya intolerance (30–50%). Some very atopic children continue to react to peptides within hydrolysed whey or casein feeds and may then respond to an amino acid based formula.

A milk-free diet (Table 9.2) involves avoidance of all cow's milk products including butter, cheese, yoghurt, and cream. It is also necessary to exclude processed foods which contain milk products or milk derivatives including casein, whey, hydrolysed whey, and non-fat milk solids. These principles also apply during weaning and care must be taken to check the ingredients listed on proprietary baby foods.

Table 9.1. Infant formulas suitable for use in CMP allergy and lactose intolerance

Soya formulas	Hydrolysed formulas
InfaSoy (Cow and Gate Nutricia)	Pepti Junior (Cow and Gate Nutricia)
Isomil (Abbot Laboratories)	
OsterSoy (Farley Health Products)	Nutramigen (Mead Johnson Nutritionals)
Prosobee (Mead Johnson Nutritionals)	Pregestimil (Mead Johnson Nutritionals)
Wysoy (SMA Nutrition)	

Table 9.2. Major foods to be excluded on a CMP free diet

Cow's milk—all types including skimmed, low fat, whole, dried, condensed, and evaporated, buttermilk

Butter, ghee, some margarines, and low fat spreads (check label)

Yoghurt, fromage frais, cream, ice cream, frozen yoghurt

Cheese, cottage cheese, cream cheese, curds

Chocolate and some other sweets may contain milk solids

Many manufactured products have milk added, avoid these ingredients listed on food labels: non-fat milk solids, whey, casein, sodium caseinate, lactoglobulin, lactalbumin

---

For additional information on suitable foods to include in a milk-free diet and milk-free manufactured products consult a State Registered Dietitian.

Under no circumstances should goats' or ewes' milk be used as infant formula as they are no less allergenic than cow's milk, contain a high solute load and are deficient in vitamins.

It is characteristic of this condition that the milk intolerance disappears after infancy usually at about 2 years of age, so that gradual re-introduction of milk containing foods and eventually milk itself should be attempted at about this time. The initial challenge should be carried out under medical supervision because of the risk of an acute anaphylactic reaction in a very small number of children.

Diagnosing food allergies

No simple and reliable diagnostic tests for suspected food intolerance are available. Skin prick tests and radio-allergosorbent tests (RAST) both of which look for specific IgE are unhelpful and not to be recommended. There are a lot of false positive tests, especially in atopic children, and false negative tests also occur. For example it is possible to have negative RAST tests and still have a severe reaction to a particular food. Detailed discussion of the indications and limitations of these methods is outside the scope of this text.

Many parents become obsessed with food allergy and try to seek help from sources where spurious pseudo-diagnostic techniques, such as hair analysis and pulse testing are employed. As a consequence they may be advised to place their children on diets which are unsound and nutritionally deficient. We have come across several children who have been advised to avoid a wide variety of foods by so-called allergy clinics, without being given necessary vitamin and mineral supplements and without proper assessment of energy needs. It can be very difficult to persuade these parents that their child is not allergic to foods and that they should revert to a normal diet. Occasionally, mistaken parental beliefs about allergy can lead to dietary restrictions severe enough to cause failure to thrive. In extreme cases this may amount to Munchausen-by-proxy, and the involvement of psychiatric services is appropriate.

Food challenges

Food challenges may be used in the initial diagnosis of food allergy and intolerance, or to confirm the diagnosis after a period of time on an exclusion diet. The best test to confirm or refute food intolerance is the double-blind placebo-controlled challenge, although in practice this is difficult to perform and remains largely a research tool. In most cases it is milk and dairy products which have been incriminated or excluded from the diet so the milk challenge is the commonest.

The introduction of milk to a child who has been adhering to a strict milk-free diet should not take place until a careful challenge has been carried out. The child is given a small quantity of milk while under medical supervision. The amount of milk ingested should gradually be increased at 20 minute intervals (Fig. 9.1), providing there is no reaction. Intramuscular adrenaline should be available in case of anaphylaxis. The exact method of the challenge varies from centre to centre. If there is a reaction the diet should be resumed and the child re-challenged at some future date. If there is no reaction a normal diet containing milk should be followed. Similar challenges can be carried out with other foods.

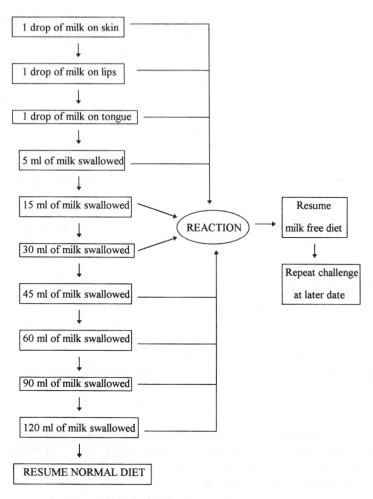

Fig. 9.1. Cow's milk challenge.

Not infrequently a child may have inadvertently been exposed to milk or other excluded foods without developing a reaction. A careful dietary history may reveal that the child has been getting supposedly excluded foods in small quantities as ingredients in manufactured products. In these circumstances, the gradual re-introduction of milk or the excluded food should take place without a formal challenge.

In many situations the ideal test is to carry out a double blind food challenge. This is particularly true where the effects are subjective or it is suspected that symptoms are being exaggerated or simulated. Blind challenges can be useful in convincing anxious parents that their child does not have a food allergy. Unfortunately they are difficult to perform because of the characteristic textures, tastes, and smells of foods. In genuinely doubtful cases they should be used despite these technical difficulties. Neither the parents, child or person administering the food should be aware of what is being ingested. If the food can be powdered and given in a capsule or disguised in a 'safe' food, the procedure is simple. It is quite easy to hide tartrazine or other food colourings, but is much more difficult when meat or fish has to be disguised or in situations where the symptoms are triggered by large quantities of food i.e. migraine.

Exclusion diets, linked with challenges if properly carried out are helpful in diagnosing food allergy. The child is started on the diet for a period of time. If the symptoms improve then other foods are gradually introduced. If the symptom recurs when a particular food has been reintroduced, then the offending food has been identified.

Dietary treatment of food intolerance

With all forms of suspected food intolerance it is important that not only is a correct diagnosis made but that careful dietary advice is given. As we have stressed in other sections of this book, children have constantly changing dietary needs and it is essential that any special diet should take this underlying progression into account and be modified with time. The elimination of food from the diet will vary in each individual child with respect to the number of foods to be excluded and how strict an exclusion is necessary. The types of food excluded may vary according to the condition being treated.

There is evidence that children whose parents perceive that they are food 'allergic' grow less well than other children. This may well be due, not so much to the effects of 'allergy' but the long term dietary imbalance which results from removing such items as milk, dairy products, and wheat from the diet without professional advice.

Exclusion diets

Exclusion diets may be used for the treatment of various forms of food intolerance. The simplest form of exclusion or elimination diet is to remove one or two foods from the diet. This can usually only be done when there is a strong suspicion that the food is the one causing the problem, for example where symptoms are worse after the child consumes cow's milk.

The first step in deciding which foods are to be excluded is to ask the family to make a record of all the foods the child eats and to note down any reactions or worsening of symptoms. This can sometimes give a clue as to which foods should be excluded and a diet based on this information should be tried for six weeks.

Another alternative is to exclude several foods which are the most likely causes of food allergy, for example milk, wheat, and eggs. The selection of foods may vary according to the condition. The advantage of the two above methods are that they involve minimal restriction of foods which tends to be easier for the family to follow. However, they do not always provide an early answer as the foods causing the problem will not necessarily have been excluded. If there is no strong suspicion as to which food or foods the child cannot tolerate, a 'full exclusion' ('oligo-antigenic', 'oligo-allergenic' or 'few foods diet') is the best approach. These terms all describe a process whereby the diet is severely restricted to a few foods. The child's intake is limited to a small number of specified foods and usually includes one meat, a milk substitute, one vegetable or family of vegetables, one fruit, one cereal, a vegetable oil, and water. The diet also sometimes includes a margarine, sugar and a low allergen drink such as colouring and preservative-free lemonade. Two examples of oligo-antigenic diets are:

- turkey, cabbage, sprouts, broccoli, cauliflower, potato, banana, soya oil, water, and salt
- lamb, carrots, parsnips, rice, pears, sunflower oil, water, and salt.

In addition, the following are required:

- vitamin and mineral supplements
- careful supervision by a dietitian
- full cooperation by parents and child.

These diets are complicated, expensive, and extremely difficult to follow so that in some cases it is advisable to start whilst the child is in hospital. It is usually recommended that the diet be followed for six weeks (Fig. 9.2). If the child's symptoms disappear then the diet should continue and a gradual reintroduction of other foods

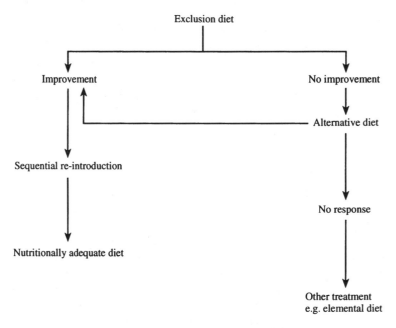

Fig. 9.2. Schema for exclusion diets.

can commence. If the child does not respond one must assume that food intolerance is not the diagnosis or that one of the foods allowed is the culprit in which case a period of elemental diet as the sole nutritional intake may be considered in very severely affected children. In our experience this is very rarely indicated.

Exclusion diets in children require careful planning by an experienced dietitian working within a team framework in an experienced paediatric unit. It may also be difficult to get the child to consume adequate energy, an important reason that the diet should only be followed for a short period of time. Food reintroduction should take place carefully and systematically. In some clinics new foods are added every two days; in others once a week. The timing will depend on the likelihood of an acute reaction. The reintroduction requires careful dietetic supervision, otherwise confusion may easily arise. The food reintroduction need not follow a specific order but it seems sensible first to reintroduce foods least likely to cause a reaction. This quickly allows the diet to become more varied and nutritionally complete. Accurate records of food intake are necessary throughout this phase and it may take six months or even a year to complete the reintroduction fully.

It is obvious that full-scale exclusion diets are major undertakings fraught with potential hazard and should be reserved for those cases where the food intolerance has major adverse effect on health.

Eczema

Eczema, or atopic dermatitis, may appear at any age and affects around 3% of children. The infantile stage begins at 2 to 6 months of age and resolves in about 50% of children by 2 to 3 years of age. It is characterized by pruritus, erythema, vesicles, exudation, and crusting. The cheeks, forehead, scalp and extensor aspects of the arms and legs are most commonly involved. The childhood stage usually occurs between 4 and 10 years of age, but may follow on from infancy and may extend into adolescence. The lesions are usually dry, scaly, itchy and well defined patches on the wrists, ankles, and in the ante-cubital and popliteal fossae. Patients with atopic dermatitis commonly have other skin abnormalities such as dry skin and goose bumps as well as a positive family history of atopic disease; 30–50% of children with atopic dermatitis will go on to develop hay fever or asthma.

Diet in eczema

Although there is a well-recognized association between atopic eczema and food intolerance, there is relatively little information available from controlled trials to show that dietary manipulation is beneficial. Exclusive breast-feeding is one way of reducing the risk of eczema, when parents are themselves atopic and the child at high risk, it may be advisable for the mother to follow a milk exclusion diet during pregnancy because of the possibility of in-utero sensitization. There is limited evidence that using a hypo-allergenic formula such as a whey or casein hydrolysate formula in the bottle-fed infant with a family history of atopy may reduce the risk of cow's milk protein intolerance and eczema, whereas soya milk does not seem to be useful in this respect. Routine 'prophylactic' use of hydrolysed protein feeds does not really appear justifiable at the present time.

Children from allergic families not already eczematous should be weaned in the normal way, but it may be prudent to avoid eggs, cow's milk, and all nuts until after the first year. Whether wheat should also be avoided is not certain unless the child is demonstrably sensitive to wheat.

In children who have already developed eczema, elimination diets may sometimes be of benefit. There are certainly some cases in which it is obvious that the ingestion of a particular food leads to an immediate flare up of the rash. Foods containing wheat, eggs, and milk have been especially associated with this type of reaction. In children in which this is so it makes practical good sense to avoid the food or foods.

Assessing the benefit of dietary change is difficult since eczema is such a fluctuating condition and in many children there is tendency to spontaneous remission with time. Psychological factors play a very important part in both the child and parents' perception of the severity of the symptoms. A state which is acceptable when all else is well can become intolerable during periods of stress.

It is against such a varying background that claims of benefit from diet manipulation have to be measured. There is at present no consensus as to the benefit of elimination diets in treating eczema. Opinion ranges from those who believe that dietary treatment is a complete waste of time and represents an example of the cure being worse than the disease, to those who would place all eczematous children on strict exclusion diets. Our view is that an oligo-antigenic diet can be justified in a very few children with intolerable symptoms unresponsive to conventional therapy, whose lives are being made so miserable by their eczema that both they and their parents are willing to put up with the considerable difficulties of an oligo-antigenic diet regimen.

Coeliac disease (gluten sensitive enteropathy)

Coeliac disease affects around 1 in 3000 children in the UK. Despite considerable geographical variation in incidence, the main trend in recent years has been a fall in the frequency of this condition. It is a permanent intolerance to dietary gluten in susceptible children, characterized by an inflammatory enteropathy of the upper small intestine causing malabsorption and failure thrive. Treatment with a gluten-free diet results in clinical and mucosal recovery and subsequent gluten challenge provokes a clinical and mucosal relapse. Most children present before the age of two years, typically with:

- failure to thrive
- anorexia
- diarrhoea
- abdominal distension
- irritability.

Older children may present atypically, for example with:

- growth failure
- iron deficiency anaemia
- delayed puberty.

The diagnosis is based on the finding of a characteristically abnormal intestinal mucosal abnormality on histological examination of a jejunal biopsy specimen. There must also be a clear cut clinical response to exclusion of gluten containing foods from the diet, preferably within several weeks. The finding of circulating antibodies in the blood (IgA antigliadin, antireticulin, and antiendomysium) at the time of diagnosis and their disappearance on gluten exclusion add weight to the diagnosis. Gluten challenge and repeat biopsy are no longer mandatory, but should be reserved for children in whom there are doubts about the initial diagnosis or adequacy of the clinical response.

The diet requires the exclusion of all gluten and gluten containing products for life. Gluten is found in wheat, rye, barley, and oats. There is some disagreement about the toxicity of oats and a recent study failed to demonstrate any abnormalities in biopsy specimens from adult coeliacs challenged with oats. Currently, however, the exclusion of oats is still recommended because long-term safety has not been established.

The diet should be based on foods known to be gluten free including meat, fish, eggs, cheese, milk, vegetables, and fruits. Many manufactured products contain gluten and care must be taken to make sure all products are gluten free. This is not always apparent from the label and it is therefore advisable to use the Coeliac Society list of manufactured foods free from gluten, or to look for the gluten-free symbol when selecting manufactured food products. There are a wide variety of special gluten-free products available, some on prescription, including gluten-free flour, bread, pasta, biscuits and cakes. The inclusion of a wide variety of gluten-free foods in the diet will ensure a nutritionally balanced diet and the child will grow at a normal rate.

The response to treatment in a classic case may be very dramatic (Fig. 9.3), but as children become older dietary compliance sometimes deteriorates. This may have potentially serious long-term consequences including linear growth faltering, and an increased risk of gastrointestinal malignancy. It is, therefore, very important that individuals with coeliac disease should continue to attend hospital clinics on a regular basis.

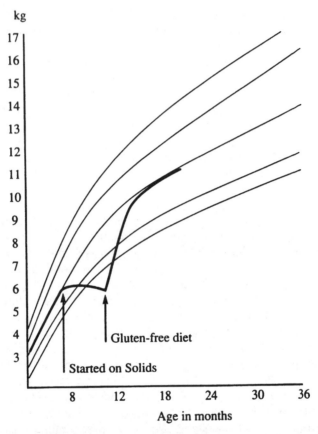

Fig. 9.3. Centile chart showing growth response of child with coeliac disease to a gluten-free diet.

Non-allergic food intolerance

Food intolerance not mediated by some disturbance of the immune mechanism may be due to untoward metabolic responses to food. There are some undoubted examples of this, such as enzyme defects, pharmacological reactions or irritant effects, but also a great deal of controversy. However, some claims of harmful effects of certain foods and their components remain unproven.

Lactose intolerance

Lactose is the carbohydrate present in all mammalian milks. Lactose intolerance results from a deficiency of the enzyme lactase which is normally present in the brush border of the enterocytes lining the small bowel. The symptoms of lactose intolerance are diarrhoea and failure to thrive with foamy, acid stools, and the presence of lactose in the stool. This can be detected simply by testing the liquid stool for reducing substances (see Chapter 7).

Very rarely lactose intolerance is present from birth (primary lactase deficiency), and would be incompatible with prolonged survival unless the infant was placed on a lactose-free formula. Secondary lactose intolerance is much more common and is seen in all conditions where there is damage to the intestinal mucosa. Thus it may occur with, or following, such diseases as gastro-enteritis, coeliac disease, or CMPI. In these conditions it is usually transient. Treatment consists of avoiding lactose containing foods until the bowel has recovered its lactase activity. Soya infant formulas contain no lactose and are suitable for this purpose provided the rest of the diet is lactose free. This is, in all respects similar to a milk-free diet but some fermented products, such as certain cheeses may in fact be lactose free and could be included in the diet. It is important to remember that some drugs may contain lactose.

Another form of lactose intolerance is seen in most racial groups other than Caucasians. This is the gradual disappearance of lactase activity from the bowel mucosa during later childhood so that in many peoples a proportion of the population is lactose-intolerant by adolescence, particularly boys. On ingestion of milk, abdominal distension, pain and diarrhoea occurs and these individuals quickly learn to avoid or limit milk or to ingest it only in a fermented form where the lactose has been converted to lactic acid. The nutritional importance of this phenomenon is that raw milk might not be a suitable dietary supplement for these older children and adolescents and that they might consequently become calcium deficient.

Migraine

Classical migraine involves unilateral headache, visual distur- bance, nausea, and vomiting, sometimes together with abdomi- nal pain. These are the end point of a number of different factors in a predisposed individual. One factor, although not usually the most important, is food intolerance. Since there are many other factors which may precipitate an attack (see Fig. 9.4) and since in some migraine sufferers food does not appear to be a factor, the response to food avoidance is very variable and often disap- pointing. In some individuals where food plays a role, other trig- gers are also present, so that food avoidance does not stop attacks altogether.

The relative importance of the role of food intolerance in migraine remains controversial. Most authorities agree that cer- tain amine-releasing foods such as cheese, citrus fruits, and chocolate may precipitate migraine attacks. Others would broad- en the range of offending substances to include many common foods and food additives notably tartrazine and an exclusion diet

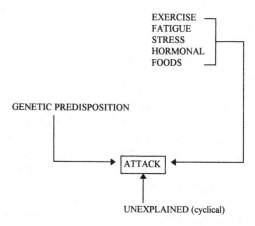

Fig. 9.4. Factors that trigger migraine.

approach similar to that for allergic conditions has been suggested. Fasting and hypoglycaemia may be an additional causative mechanism.

Dietary management of migraine

In children with severe or frequent migraine, a dietary approach to their treatment is worth considering. The first step should be to assess the child's overall nutritional intake and ensure that a well-balanced diet is being eaten, with regular meals to avoid the possibility of hypoglycaemia. This is a simple approach requiring only a few dietary changes. The next step is the elimination of those foods from the diet which may have high vaso-active amine activity. These include such foods as cheese, chocolate, and some fruit (Table 9.3).

Vaso-active agents are generally found in highest concentration in those foods which have undergone some decomposition or bacterial fermentation during their processing. Amino-acids are converted into amines which are the active agents and have long been suspected as being causes of migraine. Many adults and children will show reduction in number and severity of attacks if foods rich in vaso-active amines are removed from the diet. Foods with a high content of caffeine may also precipitate migraine symptoms and it may be sensible to avoid coffee, strong tea, and cola drinks.

Table 9.3. Foods high in vaso-active amines

Chocolate	
Yoghurt	
Cheese	
Shellfish	Smoked and pickled fish
Game	
Bananas	Citrus fruits and juices
Pineapple	Plums
Raspberries	
Peas	Broad beans
Avocado	
Yeast and meat extracts	

The diet should be adhered to for two months and become permanent if migraine attacks cease or become less frequent. Sequential reintroduction of the eliminated foods may be attempted but it may well be that it is the amount of vaso-active amine released overall rather than the effects of specific foods which is at fault. Thus foods taken in moderation may not cause an attack whereas bingeing on chocolate will exact swift retribution. Many migraine sufferers will learn for themselves what degree of avoidance is needed to keep life tolerable.

If this approach is not successful it may be appropriate to exclude other foods, particularly if any are suspected of causing attacks. In severe cases of migraine an exclusion diet may determine whether foods cause a migraine attack. A diet similar to the one discussed earlier is usually used and requires careful planning and monitoring by an experienced dietitian. Such elaborate dietary regimens are rarely worthwhile and we would not recommend them in the routine treatment of migraine as it is usually an intermittent state whereas the diet imposes continuous strain on both child and family.

Food 'allergy' in less well defined situations

Food and food additives have been blamed for a wide range of symptoms in infants and children. 'Clinical ecologists' and 'allergy specialists', many using unconventional methods of diagnosis and treatment are keen to diagnose food allergy much more readily than others. Doctors and other health professionals are often accused of being excessively sceptical about these claims and there are repeated demands from pressure groups for more allergy treatment and diagnosis to be available within the health service.

There are, however, many well founded reasons for scepticism. Most important is the fact that the claims are often based on very poor scientific foundations. Dubious investigative procedures claiming to identify presence of allergy abound, for example by hair analysis. The clinical methods employed are themselves often very suspect and advocates fail to publish their results in a way capable of proper evaluation. On these grounds alone there must be a serious question mark over the validity of the claims, but more important the justification for demands for allocation of resources to procedures based on such unsound foundations requires very careful scrutiny.

A second ground for scepticism lies in the non-specific nature of the symptoms, the fact that they are often self-limiting and are open to other explanations. For example hyperactivity in a four year old may be ascribed, among other things, to parents finding it difficult to cope with normal behaviour in a bright child, imprudent rearing practices in which the child has not been properly disciplined to accept limits to acceptable behaviour, mental or neurological handicap due to prenatal factors, and lack of stimulation or neglect. All these explanations are in varying degrees unwelcome and unpalatable and it is all too easy to blame the child's behaviour on food additives or allergy. Subjecting such a child to complex diets may aggravate the problem and lead to failure to make the correct diagnosis.

Misdiagnosis is the third important reason for healthy scepticism in this field. Particularly during infancy the risk of missing an important, treatable condition because of a wrong diagnosis of food allergy or intolerance is considerable. The authors have seen a number of such cases. It is obvious that errors of this type are potentially dangerous.

The fourth reason for scepticism is that the symptoms ascribed to food intolerance are in themselves often not a serious threat to long term health and thus the 'cure'—elaborate dieting—may be worse than the 'disease' partly because of the major inconvenience to all concerned, the considerable nutritional risks and the psychological effects of 'labelling' children with a doubtful diagnosis.

'Hyperactivity'

Since this is the most notorious example of what is usually a behaviour disturbance being ascribed to food intolerance, it deserves a section on its own. The facts are that most children diagnosed as 'hyperactive' are perfectly normal children bouncing with undirected energy. Thus most children being placed on diets for hyperactivity have other explanations for their behaviour. Furthermore the evidence that there is a subgroup of hyperactive children who might benefit from additive-free diets remains very dubious. Independent double blind studies have failed to reveal benefit while anecdotal claims of response in individual children are open to all the usual criticisms in situations where there are often powerful psychological factors at work and where the symptoms are likely to resolve with time anyway.

Health care workers find themselves in some difficulties in this and similar situations. Many parents have become thoroughly convinced that the diet is to blame for their children's problems, a premise often given undue prominence in the media. Advocates of 'unconventional methods' feel none of the inhibitions against outrageous public pronouncements and totally unsubstantiated claims which make headlines and which are so difficult to counter, and no obligation to subject their claims to scientific scrutiny.

Many children, as in the case of those being treated for allergy are put onto diets on the advice of 'self-help' groups or professionals with little knowledge or understanding of children's nutritional needs. Since many of the 'conditions' being treated are not organic or are self-limited or are in the minds of the parents rather than the bodies of their children, it is not difficult for such practitioners or their dubious methods to chalk up 'successes' when all others have 'failed' or have 'refused to recognize the true nature' of the complaint. This is a growing and worrying problem for which there is no obvious immediate solution. Health workers are on a hiding to nothing in attempting to deal with such cases. If they refuse to become involved, the child may suffer serious nutritional harm. If they assist the parents to maintain diets for non-existent diseases they are perpetuating the evil. When such families are encountered there is a responsibility to help the parents to find a rational solution to their children's difficulties or at very least to ensure that their diets are adequate.

Although there is no strong evidence to implicate artificial colouring agents and other additives there is no reason why processed foods which contain them should not be eliminated from the diet. Not all so-called E numbers are artificial agents and many have been included in foods from time immemorial. The E-numbers are given to a list of food additives drawn up by the European Community which are generally regarded as safe for use. They include naturally occurring colourants, gums, vitamins, and preservatives. Examples of these are given in Table 9.4. There are certain groups of E-numbers particularly artificial colours and preservatives which may be suspect and are probably well avoided. These include the well-known colouring agents E 102 (tartrazine) and E 110 (sunset yellow); both are azo dyes. Preservatives include the benzoate group E 210–219. Both the azo dyes and benzoates have been known to cause asthmatic attacks in susceptible individuals. Their effects on behaviour are less well documented. However, they are fairly easy to avoid, and unnecessary additions to the diet. A diet based largely on fresh, unprocessed foods is more likely to meet healthy eating recommendations.

Table 9.4. Examples of natural and permitted additives

Colours	
Caramel (brown)	E 150
Riboflavin (yellow)	E 101
Chlorophyll (green)	E 140
Carbon (black)	E 153
Alpha carotene (Yellow, orange)	E 160 (a)
Preservative	
Acetic acid	E 260
Lactic acid	E 270
Anti-oxidants	
Ascorbic acid and derivatives	E 300–305
Tocopherols	E 306–309
Emulsifiers and stabilizers	
Citric acid and its derivatives	E 330–333
Agar	E 406
Pectin	E 440

Further reading

Caffarelli, C., Terzi, V., Perrone, F., and Cavaghi, G., (1996). Food related, exercise induced anaphylaxis. *Arch. Dis. Child*, **75**, 141–4.

Chandra, R.K., Puri, A., and Hamed, A. (1989). Influence of maternal diet during lactation and use of formula feeds on development of atopic eczema in high risk infants. *British Medical Journal*, **229**, 228–30.

David, T.J. (1995). Food intolerance. In *Nutrition in Child Health* (ed. D.P. Davies), pp.165–78. Royal College of Physicians of London, London.

Ferguson, A. (1992). Definitions and diagnosis of food intolerance and food allergy: consensus and controversy. *Journal of Pediatrics*, **121**, S7–S11.

Høst, A. (ed.) (1994). Cow's milk protein allergy and intolerance in infancy. *Pediatric Allergy and Immunology*, **5**, (Supplement 5).

Hourihane, J.O'B., Dean, T.P., and Warner, J.O., (1996). Peanut allergy in relation to heredity, maternal diet, and other atopic diseases; results of a questionnaire survey, skin prick testing, and food challenges. *British Medical Journal*, **313**, 518–21.

Sampson, H.A. (1996). Managing peanut allergy. *British Medical Journal*, (editorial), **312**, 1050–1.

10

....

Obesity

Obesity is associated with a greatly increased likelihood of diabetes, hypertension, hyperlipidaemia, and heart disease in adult life as well as increased rates of breast, colon, and uterine cancer. In the UK 13% of men and 16% of women are now considered obese, double the number in 1980 and it is highly probable that this trend will also be found in children. Obesity can be viewed as a maladaptive increase in the size of the adipose organ, the amount of adipose tissue in the body reflecting the cumulative balance between energy intake and output (Fig. 10.1). In the individual, obesity may result from a disorder of energy intake, output, or both. Obesity has become more common in the UK despite the fact that average energy intake has declined. The implication is that levels of physical activity, and hence energy needs, have declined even faster.

The health of the nation initiative has recognized obesity as a key target and has set goals for a substantial reduction by the year 2005. Targeting obese children for weight reduction seems logical since fat children tend to become fat adults. In practice, however, effective treatment (achieving appropriate weight for height and age) often proves extremely difficult and calls into question the justification for such a selective strategy. Despite

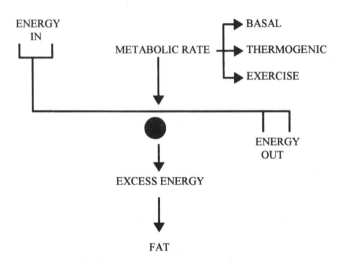

Fig. 10.1. Energy balance and obesity.

this, even some reduction of fat is probably still worthwhile and may improve self image as well as reduce later morbidity.

Prevalence of obesity

There are large differences in estimates of the prevalence of obesity in children. One problem is that there is no universally accepted definition which differentiates between fatness without medical implications and fatness that is medically undesirable. Obesity appears to be more common in the United States than elsewhere in the world and affects as many as 25% of children and 30% of the adult population, contributing around 8% of all illness costs. In the UK, detailed surveys of 11–12 year old children in Newcastle in 1990 showed that children had become heavier for their height than a decade earlier despite a general reduction in energy intake, once again suggesting a decrease in the general level of physical activity. In all countries children from poor socio-economic backgrounds seem to have a greater prevalence of obesity.

Causes of obesity

The 'common sense' view that obesity is caused by overeating is widely held yet difficult to substantiate. Moreover, it is a circular argument, since only the individual who is fat can be said to have overeaten. It now seems likely that the body has a complex, highly sophisticated system for regulating fat stores, although the details of how this control mechanism actually operates are not yet fully understood.

Environmental

The evidence that environmental factors have a role in the causation of obesity is borne out by many studies which show that obesity is, at least to some extent, determined by life-style and eating habits. Sedentary populations on high calorie intakes have a greater incidence of obesity. In some communities, changing social patterns or emigration have resulted in dramatic changes in degree of adiposity. Sex differences and reversals of relative obesity at certain ages also indicate that there are very important environmental effects on the amount of fat accumulated.

The physical activity, or lack of it in modern western children caused by changes in life-style may well be a contributing factor to the increases in childhood obesity. Obese children are probably less physically fit than lean children but it is not clear whether this is cause or effect.

The amount of television children watch is said to be an important contributory factor to obesity and in the United States children spend on average as much time watching television as attending school. TV watching is often associated with the intake of high fat, high carbohydrate snacks and drinks, a pattern encouraged by the advertisements between the programmes. Television watching therefore combines high energy intake with low energy expenditure and possibly a reduction in metabolic rate. Perhaps the association is indirect since children who are fat may shun or be shunned by other children and be forced into excessive television watching. Other possible causes include the lack of safe places for children to play in large cities so that they stay indoors. There has also been an increase in sedentary video and computer games with a reduction in priority given to physical education at schools. It may be that as with a general increase in energy intake, a general decline in physical activity causes obesity in those children who are genetically predisposed to accumulate adipose tissue. There is probably a vicious cycle in which children who get fat because of a combination of inactivity and excessive food intake become even more inactive.

Genetic

Family studies demonstrate that parents who are overweight tend to have children who are overweight and that two overweight parents are even more likely to have overweight offspring. The similarity of body habitus amongst family members and the high correlation between weight for height and skinfold thickness between identical twins argue in favour of a major genetic contribution to obesity. For example the body mass index (BMI) of adopted children is much more strongly associated with BMI of their biological parents than that of their adoptive parents.

Recently a team of investigators studying the genetics of obesity has succeeded both in characterizing an obesity gene in mice, and finding a DNA region in the human that is 84% identical to the mouse gene. The gene product has now been isolated and termed 'leptin' from the Greek *leptos* meaning thin. Defective production of leptin in adipose cells results in gross obesity in the obese mouse. Leptin is taken up by the brain and possibly leads to a decrease in the concentration of a neuropeptide that stimulates food intake. In another mouse model, it is a defect in the receptor for leptin that appears to lead to obesity. So far, no case of obesity in man has been found to result from a defect in the leptin producing gene, but increased linkage to the gene has been found in massively obese individuals. In addition, the capacity to transport leptin into the brain is lower in obese individuals and may be the mechanism for leptin resistance.

Genetic – environmental interactions

Whereas genetic and metabolic factors may determine which children are most at risk of becoming fat, it could be that it is the general pattern of eating and exercise which determines how many individuals will actually become overweight. It is also possible that individuals with an extreme risk of obesity will get fat on quite low energy intakes. In others the amount eaten may be the crucial factor in determining whether they become fat. All clinicians will have had experience of patients who have been fat at some time in their lives but who subsequently lose their overweight. One would not expect this to happen if the degree of adiposity was entirely genetically and metabolically determined. It has been estimated that around four out of five obese people could lose weight if they lived in a less fatness-promoting environment, whilst perhaps one in five may be genetically obese in the sense that would probably remain fat even in an environment that promoted leanness.

Psychological factors

While this is not the place to discuss the very complex neurological and psychological factors which determine eating behaviour there are some aspects of this fascinating area which are of general interest.

The basic mechanisms which underlie the process of eating are located in the hypothalamus of the brain which contains centres both for hunger and satiety, responsive to a variety of stimuli (Fig. 10.2). In man there are powerful cognitive factors which after infancy may override the more primitive visceral responses.

It was thought for a time that obesity was due to overeating secondary to a mismatch or misinterpretation of so-called eating cues. External cues are stimuli such as the appearance, smell, or taste of food, whereas internal cues are the sensations normally interpreted as hunger or satiation. These ideas have become the basis for much behaviour modification management.

One valuable concept, that of restrained and unrestrained eaters has emerged. A restrained eater is an individual who

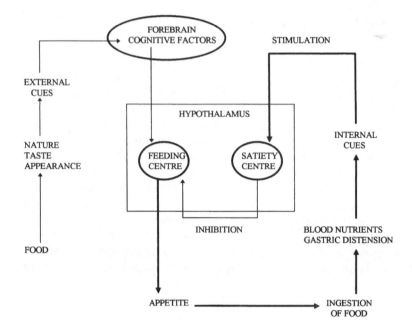

Fig. 10.2. Effects of various stimuli on the eating process.

consciously or unconsciously, as a result of conditioning, limits the amount of food ingested below complete satiation, whereas an unrestrained eater ingests to the point of complete satiation. Most individuals who become restrained eaters may have a fear or distaste for becoming obese. The extreme end of this spectrum may be anorexia nervosa.

Young children are by nature unrestrained eaters but peer pressures force at least some to control the amount they ingest. Parents who are themselves restrained eaters may ensure that their children do not eat to the point where they become obese. These factors may explain how some families with the genetic potential for obesity remain lean, whereas others succumb to their genes.

The dietary intake of an obese person may vary from low to high in different states of adiposity. Someone who has just lost weight from a diet may eat voraciously if unrestrained until the body returns to its accustomed state of fatness. Some mechanism may then act on the internal cue system to reduce the amount ingested. An obese individual may be restraining food intake once obese, so that no further increase in adiposity occurs, but insufficiently to lose weight. In both situations the diet will be normal or even low in energy. Some lean people with high metabolic rate may be unrestrained eaters but on the other hand some lean people are only lean by virtue of the fact that they are restraining their dietary intake.

Consequences of childhood obesity

During childhood

There is a significant social stigma associated with being obese. Fat people are the victims of prejudice and discrimination since it is generally perceived that to be fat is somehow 'unhealthy' and the fat person is guilty of both sloth and gluttony. Studies in the USA have shown that overweight adolescents are less likely to marry, and more likely to have low household incomes than those who have not been overweight. School children suffer teasing and torment at the hands of both peers and teachers, yet diet is for some an even worse alternative. Most obese individuals are not emotionally disturbed although adolescents may have a poor image of themselves and become depressed. This may be a result of futile attempts to slim.

Gross or 'morbid' obesity is rare in children. Those pathological conditions predisposing to obesity usually present with short stature or other symptoms before obesity becomes a major problem. Such conditions include the following:

- endocrine   hypothyroidism
                           Cushing's syndrome
                           craniopharyngioma
- 'hypothalamic'   Prader–Willi syndrome
                           Laurence–Moon–Biedl syndrome

- chromosomal   Down syndrome
                        Klinefelter's syndrome
- drug treatment   corticosteroids
- reduced activity   spina bifida

It is among this group of children that harmful or potentially life-threatening problems, such as orthopaedic complications, Pickwickian Syndrome (alveolar-hypoventilation) or cardiomyopathy can be expected to occur. These problems are very rare in children who are merely plump and their prevalence should not be exaggerated.

Long-term effects

Although the statistical association between obesity and vascular disease seems to be beyond question, it is by no means certain that there is a direct causal relationship. When other risk factors such as hypertension and abnormal lipid patterns are excluded, obesity on its own does not appear to be very strongly associated with morbidity. On the other hand strong correlation exists with high LDL-cholesterol, low HDL-cholesterol and hypertension which are all undoubted risk factors for vascular disease.

Should childhood obesity be treated?

With regards to the population as a whole, the most practical anti-obesity intervention is to modify the environment in terms of habitual physical activity and food intake. What is to be done with children who are already fat? Young fat children whose food intakes are determined by their parents can be made to lose weight by 'involuntary dieting' but anyone who has tried to cope with older 'free-range' children will be aware of the difficulties involved in maintaining weight loss. The child must genuinely wish to become thinner, and obese parents must be willing to change their eating habits and lose weight themselves.

Which children should be considered for dietary treatment?

Given that most obese children placed on diets fail to maintain permanent weight loss there is a good case for a selective approach. The trouble is that often both remaining fat and submitting to draconian diets are equally unacceptable. Little wonder that obesity has been labelled the 'miserable condition'. In some situations, a more positive stance is indicated. Children with a family history of vascular disease or diabetes are particularly at risk and it is legitimate to warn of the health hazards. Similarly, children with a genuinely raised blood pressure or with a family history of hypertension should have firmer advice. Care needs to be taken in interpreting blood pressure readings in overweight children because false high readings are common. Children presenting themselves for weight reduction are worth an effort but even here, the proportion of failures remains high.

Dietary treatment

The ideal is to prevent obesity in the first place and emphasis should be placed on healthy eating and exercise for the whole family, along with establishing good food habits in early childhood. Treatment of childhood obesity using dietary manipulation would appear simple; however, in practice it can be extremely difficult. Children find it difficult to follow dietary regimens which set them apart form other children, they need a great deal of support from their families. If overweight parents are unwilling to change their dietary habits it is unlikely that the overweight child will change his or her eating habits.

Very low calorie liquid diets (less than 600 kcal) are popular among the obese adult population and are advertised and marketed in every health food shop and newspaper. They claim to promote rapid weight loss. We do not wish to discuss the pitfalls of these diets in relation to adults but must stress that they are not suitable for infants and children and can lead to nutritional deficiencies and poor growth. Liquid diets do not promote a long-term healthy eating pattern which is necessary for children to remain stable after weight loss.

Another category of very low calorie diets are based on 'normal' foods and aim to provide very low energy intakes for example 300, 400, or 600 kcal daily. These are also unsuitable for children. The low energy intake makes it virtually impossible for the child to consume adequate protein, vitamins, and minerals and long-term use will certainly impair a child's growth. It should be noted that these diets are very inflexible, unpalatable, and difficult to follow.

Other forms of dietary treatment include the many different 'fad diets' such as the 'F' plan, Scarsdale, egg, grapefruit, or Mars Bar diets. They have transient notoriety with often exaggerated claims for their effectiveness. However, some are well balanced and with slight modification can be suitable for children but others are not acceptable. Before considering one of these diets for a child a careful assessment must be made to ensure that it provides a good nutritional balance. The overall energy should not be less than 1000 kcal and as previously discussed, care must be taken when giving high-fibre diets to young children.

A sensible, healthy eating plan consisting of low energy but high nutrient dense foods is preferable to any of the above. Calorie counting is not usually necessary although it can be a good way of avoiding excess and achieving a balanced diet. General guidelines for reducing a child's energy intake and maintaining a healthy, balanced diet include:

- limit intake of fried foods, high energy, low nutrient dense snack foods, and concentrated sugary foods
- remove all visible fat from meat and choose low fat meat products
- eat only at meal times and recognized snack times
- substitute fresh fruit for puddings
- replace high sugar squash and fizzy drinks with low calorie counterparts
- substitute semi-skimmed or skimmed milk for whole milk, include a minimum of 300 ml and a maximum of 600 ml daily
- use butter or margarine sparingly or preferably a low fat spread
- use low fat cream cheese, yoghurt, and fromage frais in place of full fat products and cream.

An example of suitable dietary guidelines for children wishing to lose weight is shown in Fig. 10.3 with a sample of a menu plan in Table 10.1. Families will require further information regarding suitable cereal and protein exchanges, low calorie recipes, snack and packed lunch ideas. If the child usually has a school lunch the school will need to be contacted and a suitable meal requested.

If a strict regimen is necessary and the child's food intake falls below 1000 calories, vitamin and mineral supplements should be given. All children on dietary restriction should be monitored carefully to ensure that their overall nutrition and growth is not impaired.

Table 10.1. Sample menu plan based on Fig. 10.3

Breakfast	small glass of unsweetened fruit juice wholegrain cereal, milk from allowance and/or wholemeal toast with margarine tea or coffee, milk from allowance, no sugar
Mid-morning snack	fresh fruit (if wanted) low-calorie squash
Lunch	lean meat or fish vegetables or salad fresh fruit or low-calorie yoghurt low-calorie squash or water
Mid-afternoon snack	cup of tea or low-calorie squash or fizzy drink 1 slice wholemeal toast with margarine
Evening meal	lean meat or cheese or egg vegetables or salad 1 small portion of boiled potato fresh fruit or unsweetened canned fruit low-calorie squash or drink of milk from daily allowance
Bed-time snack	tea or low-calorie squash wholemeal toast or wholegrain cereal if allowances permit

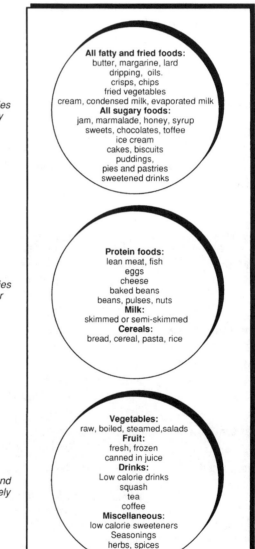

STOP

High in calories to be strictly limited or avoided

STEADY

Quite high in calories but necessary for growth. Daily allowances recommended

GO

Low in calories and can be eaten freely

Fig. 10.3. Traffic light guide to healthy food choices for a healthy weight.

Bear in mind the following points:

* drastic weight losing programmes may affect linear growth
* dramatic initial weight loss may be due to loss of lean body mass
* aim for a gradual weight loss, or maintenance of a stable weight
* encourage graduated exercise.

Exercise is a very important factor in helping a child to lose weight. Children should be encouraged to participate in the usual school sports and games, as well as take up some other forms of exercise out of school. Some obese children are reluctant to take part in sport because of their appearance and in some cases it may help to start weight reduction with a home-based exercise programme initially. This will be more effective if undertaken with other family members. Exercise should be graduated and this can begin with walking instead of travelling by bus or car. It is important that exercise is taken at least three times a week and continues for a sufficiently long period. Short bursts of exercise are anaerobic and do not burn fat. Aerobic exercise will burn fat and increase metabolic rate during exercise and possibly for some time afterwards. Exercise will not only assist weight loss but will also promote a feeling of well-being. Children following a weight reducing program benefit from:

* a great deal of support and regular follow-up
* follow-up outside of hospital (school or local health clinic)
* group sessions, which help some but not all.

The overweight infant should be dealt with in a completely different way. Strict dietary regimens are not appropriate for the child under the age of one year and probably not before two years. Simple modifications should be made to the feeding pattern and some alterations in the types of foods offered, the emphasis being on a gradual introduction of a healthy diet as outlined in the weaning section of Chapter 2.

Suggestions for modifying the feeds of the overweight baby, weanling, and toddler include:

* infant formula should not be over concentrated.

- a feeding plan which gives appropriate times and volumes of feed
- use a small hole teat to slow down rate of ingestion
- give water rather than more milk when thirsty
- sugar and solids must not be added to bottle feeds.

Weaning should be started at an appropriate age, not before 4–6 months. Low energy dense solids foods with a high nutrient content should be given in preference to high energy dense solids. Examples of these include puréed fruit, vegetables, wholegrain cereals, and lean meats. It is also helpful to avoid prolonged use of a bottle and a cup should be introduced from about six or seven months of age.

Behaviour modification

Attempts to alter the eating patterns of children has led to the development of behaviourally-based strategies which have had varying success. Most include:

- positive reinforcement (rewards)
- ensuring that participants understand the material presented to them
- record keeping by parents and children of weight, food intake, and their reactions to meals
- provision of ideal eating models for the rest of the family
- agreeing a contract with parents.

Acquiring self-management skills using congitive behaviour modification methods are relatively more successful in older children, whereas parental management is more important in the younger ones. Behaviour modification programs have been used in the school setting, within obesity clinics, and as a component of family-based programs.

Family-Based treatment

Family-based systems are based on observations that children lost similar amounts of weight during the initial phases of weight reducing schedules, but those in whom the parents had been involved showed a more sustained response. There are three essential components to the treatment programme:

- diet using the 'traffic light' system
- an exercise programme
- behavioural treatment programme for parents and older children.

The child is expected to keep a written record of the various foods ingested in their appropriate categories. Parents are expected to praise children for keeping to the restrictions of the various categories of foods.

Preventing childhood obesity

No one can doubt that it is a disadvantage to be overweight whether or not it is a significant risk factor for subsequent disease. There seems to be a strong case for discouraging young children from becoming overweight if this can be achieved. Those who believe that obesity is largely genetically determined may regard this as impossible. We prefer the view that some children will benefit if the overall adiposity of the population can be prevented from rising by sensible policies, even if some individuals very strongly predisposed to obesity will get fat irrespective of environmental factors. Repeating the experience of the United States, where there appears to be an explosion of obesity among both children and adults is something we must try to avoid.

It was thought that infantile obesity programmed individuals to a lifetime of being overweight, events during the first months of life probably have little bearing on later body habitus, provided that the infant is fed either breast milk or correctly prepared infant formula and not commenced on high calorie solids too early. Most very plump infants slim down during early childhood and true infantile obesity persisting into adulthood is very rare. Apart from following the laid down principles for infant feeding, there seems little justification for the introduction of policies aimed at preventing overweight in babies.

Much more important seems to be the post-toddler period. The age period from two years to six years is the leanest time of life, so the onset of obesity during this time is an important matter which may have a permanent effect. Significant obesity begins to appear in the preschoolchild. Just why some children not previously fat begin to put on weight is not really understood. Metabolically based theories do not explain this, as one would expect individuals predetermined to be fat to be so from the start. It seems prudent to assume that the pattern of eating and activity has something to do with it.

This is the period where children may adopt particular patterns of eating and physical activity. Parents who find it convenient to place a child in front of a television or video screen with a bag of crisps and a bottle of pop should be aware that this is an unsound practice with possible long-term harmful consequences. Social policy which leads to the trapping of families into this sort of life-style needs to be re-examined.

Parents should be encouraged to avoid excessive calorie and fat intakes in their children's diets and to discourage snacking on 'empty calorie' foods and drinks. If parents are overweight they should be encouraged to re-examine thier own eating and activity patterns. The promotion of a life-style for the whole family which involves a reasonable amount of physical activity is to be encouraged. Regrettably UK National Travel Surveys have demonstrated a decline of about 20% in annual distance walked, and 27% in distance cycled between 1985 and 1993. A recent strategy statement from the Department of Health highlights the need to promote moderate activity in children as a priority; however, encouraging children to walk or cycle to school is unlikely to be successful unless they can do this in a safe environment.

The prevalence of obesity increases sharply after adolescence and goes on increasing into adult life. Paradoxically some fat children may slim down during adolescence, presumably because of cognitive pressures. Many simply decide that they will not be fat any longer. A population of 'restrained eaters' emerges, people who consciously or unconsciously restrain their intake of energy to achieve a desirable body habitus but who would, presumably because of the nature of their genetically determined metabolism, become obese otherwise. This subset of the population at least demonstrates that some individuals can alter their body weight by dietary means.

Further reading

Caro, J.F., Kolaczynski, J.W., Nyce, M.R., Ohannesian, J.P., Opentanoval, I., Goldman, W.H., Lynn, R.B., Zhang, P.L., Sinha, M.K., and Considine, R.U. (1996). Decreased cerebrospinal-fluid/serum leptin ratio in obesity: a possible mechanism for leptin resistance. *Lancet,* **348**, 159–61.

Dietz, W.H., and Gortmaker, S.L. (1985). Do we fatten our children at the television set? Obesity and television viewing in children and adolescents. *Pediatrics,* **75**, 807–12.

Editorial (1992). Born to be fat? *Lancet,* **340**, 881–2.

Hassink, S.G., Sheslow, D.V., deLancey, E., Opentanova, I., Considine, R.V., and Caro, J.F. (1996). Serum leptin in children with obesity: relationship to gender and development. *Pediatrics,* **98**(2), 201–3.

Poskitt, E.M.E. (1987). Management of obesity. *Archives of Disease in Childhood,* **62**, 305–10.

11

··

Dietary management of metabolic disorders

Special diets play an important role in the management of a number of diseases. They need careful planning, have to be tailored to the individual needs of the patient, and long-term clinical and biochemical monitoring is necessary to ensure adequate nutrition. Here we provide a basic outline of the principles which underlie their management. The diets are complicated and should be carried out by a specialist team including a paediatrician, paediatric dietitian, specialist nurse and where appropriate, a biochemist with expertise in the field. In some conditions other health workers should be part of the team, for example physiotherapists in cystic fibrosis. Ideally outpatient consultations should be carried out jointly by all members of the team.

Regular, careful measurement and assessment of physical and intellectual development is a cornerstone of successful management. The most important evidence that the diet is satisfactory, is the growth of the child. The emotional needs of families (including siblings) with children on special and complicated diets may be considerable, requiring much community support by specially trained personnel. Wherever possible a health visitor or nurse practitioner should be attached to the laboratory and/or clinic, seeing the family with the paediatrician and acting as a liaison between the central service and the community. Such a person can be of enormous benefit in the guidance of health professionals and education service regarding the needs of the child. By regular visits to the home, better control of diet is often possible, misunderstandings can be resolved and by providing a link between families and various parts of the service, an esprit de corps may be created that is not otherwise easy to achieve. The brothers and sisters of children on diets may feel neglected and their needs must be actively considered. If possible they should be made to feel part of the team.

A hospital-based social worker who attends the special clinic can acquire a very useful understanding of the problems of these often stressed families and may be of great assistance in easing their difficulties. Ideally dietitians should be ready to make home visits regularly. Unfortunately constraints on resources do not always allow for this. Nevertheless the occasional visit can be enormously beneficial.

All this expertise and experience can only be attained if there is a reasonable concentration of patients. In some rare disorders cases may be scattered over a wide area. It is highly desirable for many reasons that all such children should be seen from time to time at the specialist centre. Management of some conditions is evolving all the time. There are constant changes in what is regarded as 'best practice' which passes along the grape-vine and will not be known to most doctors and dietitians. New products which make diets easier to cope with are produced regularly. Parents with children on unusual diets being treated away from specialist centres often complain that they are not kept abreast of such developments.

Dealing with many cases gives the specialist paediatricians and dietitians a 'feel' they would not otherwise possess. The furtherance of knowledge, which most parents would wish to see also requires some concentration of cases.

Unfortunately there is sometimes a reluctance to part with what are regarded as 'interesting cases'. A team approach to management is the essence of success. This is emphatically not an area for the 'rugged individualist' consultant paediatrician giving orders to others. We have seen many examples of children receiving less than optimal care because of this. Some form of 'shared care' system may be evolved between the local paediatrician and dietetic service and the specialist unit. Parents of children with rare diseases have a right to be referred to specialist centres.

Inborn errors of metabolism

Of those inborn errors of metabolism which are amenable to treatment, dietary management is crucial to almost all. In many cases this involves eliminating or reducing from the diet some component of normal nutrition which cannot be properly metabolized. (e.g. phenylalanine in phenylketonuria). In others it is a matter of supplementing the diet with a nutrient that may be deficient as a consequence of the enzyme defect (e.g. glucose in acyl-CoA-dehydrogenase defects). A third group of disorders are those in which the requirements for certain vitamins or enzyme co-factors are greatly increased and huge doses of normal vitamins may be needed (e.g. biotin in biotinidase deficiency). This last group is particularly rewarding because effective treatment with a dietary agent is so simple and effective (see Fig. 11.1). In a fourth group of inborn disorders, diet plays a supportive and very important role in management (e.g. cystic fibrosis).

Prevalence

Individually, treatable inborn errors of metabolism are not common, but taken as a group they constitute a significant number of children with potential handicap, morbidity, and mortality. For each million people in the population there will be born each year about 30 children with a genetic disorder likely to benefit from dietary help (Table 11.1). With passage of time more conditions at present untreatable may become at least in part amenable to dietary management.

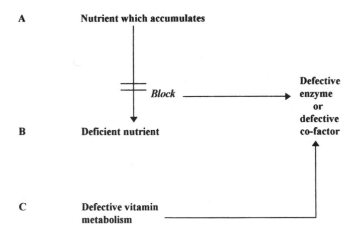

A: restrict nutrient, i.e. phenylalanine in phenylketonuria (PKU), phenylalanine and tyrosine in tyrosinemia, isoleucine, leucine and valine in Maple Syrup Urine disease, galactose in galactosaemia.

B: provide extra nutrient, i.e. tyrosine in PKU, cystine in homocystinuria.

C: give large doses of vitamin, i.e. biotin in biotinidase deficiency, cobalamin in cobalamin transport disorders.

Fig. 11.1. Inborn errors of metabolism.

Table 11.1. Frequency of genetic disorders amenable to dietary treatment

Disease	Incidence
Hyperlipidaemia Type IIa	1 in 500
Cystic fibrosis	1 in 2500
Phenylketonuria	1 in 10 000
Other inborn errors	1 in 10 000

Hyperlipidaemia

Lipids (fats) exist in the body as triglycerides, cholesterol, and phospholipids and are transported bound to specific proteins. These are known as lipoproteins and incorporate different amounts of cholesterol and triglyceride and have different functions. The two main types of primary hyperlipidaemia encountered in childhood are Type IIa familial hypercholesterolaemia in which the LDL cholesterol is increased in the blood, and Type I or familial lipoprotein lipase deficiency where there is an increase in chylomicrons. Type IIa hyperlipidaemia is by far the most common inherited metabolic disorder, Type I being a much rarer condition.

Type IIa hyperlipidaemia (hypercholesterolaemia)

Type IIa hypercholesterolaemia is an autosomal dominant inherited disorder occurring in the homozygous and the heterozygous forms. The latter being the more common with an incidence of 1:500 in the population. It is characterized by raised serum cholesterol levels, most significantly, LDL-cholesterol is elevated from a very early age. As a consequence, the condition is associated with a high incidence of premature ischaemic heart disease. Early diagnosis and treatment can prevent this.

Children at risk include those from families where there is a history of someone having a heart attack at an early age or someone with a known raised serum cholesterol. Not all hypercholesterolaemia is due to this inherited defect. Most adults with raised LDL-cholesterol do not have type IIa hyperlipidaemia. Nevertheless all children who have a parent or grandparent, aunt or uncle who developed early cardio-vascular disease should be screened for hyperlipidaemia. If their serum cholesterol is raised they should follow a diet with:

- reduced overall fat content to 30–35 % of energy
- saturated fat limited to 10 % of energy
- polyunsaturated fat to provide no more than 10 % of energy
- monounsaturated fat to provide the balance, usually 10–12 % energy

- increase carbohydrate, especially complex carbohydrate, intake to meet energy needs
- foods high in soluble NSP such as oats, beans, and pulses, have a cholesterol lowering effect and should be encouraged along with a wide variety of foods.

Experience so far suggests that children and adolescents require careful dietary follow-up by an experienced paediatric dietitian to make sure that the diets are nutritionally adequate and normal growth occurs. Success with diet has been shown to be more effective where regular follow-up and family support is provided. Long-term management generally requires a combination of diet and drug treatment. The drug treatment of choice in children is usually cholestyramine or colestipol. These drugs bind bile salts in the intestinal tract preventing their re-absorption and therefore the re-absorption of cholesterol. Parent support groups are very helpful in improving motivation.

It is important that the diet is followed for life and serum cholesterol levels are checked regularly as a way of monitoring dietary compliance. It is often difficult for a child to follow such a diet if the rest of the family eat differently. Dietary advice should be aimed at the whole family as the diet, which follows the COMA recommendations, will certainly not harm unaffected members.

Because individuals with type IIa hypercholesterolaemia survive well into adult life it is possible for them to have children. In 1 in 250 000 families both parents will carry the abnormal gene. A quarter of their children will thus inherit two abnormal genes for the condition and be homozygous. This is a devastating state which responds poorly to diet and leads to death from myocardial infarction in the second or third decade. Treatment includes plasmaphoresis and small bowel by-pass. Fortunately, it is extremely rare, about two cases per million births.

Type I hyperlipidaemia

Type I lipoprotein lipase deficiency is an extremely rare autosomal recessive disorder. The basic defect is a deficiency of lipoprotein lipase which hydrolyses dietary triglycerides or apolipoprotein C-II deficiency which results in a failure to activate lipoprotein lipase. This causes a failure to clear chylomicrons at a normal rate. In infants and young children the clinical presentation includes attacks of abdominal pain, eruptive xanthoma (skin lesions), and hepatosplenomegaly. The serum is milky in the fasting state with a gross elevation of triglyceride (neutral fats). The treatment is a very low fat diet with increased carbohydrate to ensure adequate energy intake. Medium chain triglycerides (MCT) can also be used to increase energy and more importantly to make the diet more palatable. MCT is usually used as an oil for frying or coating foods. When absorbed it does not form chylomicrons. As with all severely fat restricted diets the child's intake of fat soluble vitamins will be low and supplements of vitamin A, D, E, and K are necessary.

Cystic fibrosis

Cystic fibrosis (CF) is the commonest major autosomal recessive disorder found in Caucasian populations in the western world. The incidence in Britain is approximately 1:2500 live births. It affects boys and girls equally. It is a multi-organ disorder with widespread dysfunction of the exocrine and mucus-secreting glands, characterized by chronic pulmonary disease, pancreatic insufficiency, liver dysfunction, and abnormally high sweat electrolytes. The CF gene was cloned in 1989 and many different mutations have now been identified and probably account for the varying clinical features of the disease.

Approximately 10% of children with CF present with meconium ileus at birth. The remainder are identified in early childhood with recurrent chest infections, failure to thrive, abdominal pain, and malabsorption. The diagnosis is confirmed by a raised concentration of sodium and chloride in the sweat on at least two tests. The immuno-reactive trypsin (IRT) test is used for screening (raised in CF) and is routinely performed in some centres. Antenatal diagnosis is also possible.

The main problem in cystic fibrosis is respiratory disease. Severe chronic lung infection leads to a gradual deterioration in pulmonary function in most children. Malnutrition has adverse effects on lung function and maintaining good nutrition has been shown to delay deterioration in lung function and improve growth and therefore survival rates.

Nutritional problems are multifactorial and include malabsorption related to the insufficiency of pancreatic enzymes, poor appetite with inadequate food intake, increased requirements due to recurrent infection, and urinary glucose losses due to diabetes.

The problems of malabsorption can be largely overcome by the use of enteric coated pancreatic enzyme supplements such as pancrease and creon which are extremely effective. The enzymes need to be taken with all food. Larger amounts are necessary with meals and smaller ones with snacks. Excessive intakes of pancreatic enzymes have been associated with colonic strictures in a small group of children and high dose lipase preparations are no longer recommended.

Nutritional requirements of children with cystic fibrosis include:

- increased energy intake to 120–150 % of average requirements
- a normal to high fat intake
- increased protein intake
- fat soluble vitamin supplements
- salt supplements in hot weather.

To achieve these increases, dietary supplements are usually necessary and in some cases supplementary tube feedings may be used (see Chapter 12). Because of the growing complexity of management and the problematic nature of some current therapy, children may require repeated stays in hospital. The treatment including the administration of antibiotics, enzyme preparations, dietary supplements, and physiotherapy take up a great deal of time. The families need much help and support. The Cystic Fibrosis Research Trust offers support and advice.

Phenylketonuria

Phenylketonuria is an autosomal recessive disorder with an incidence of 1:10 000 births in Britain. It results from a deficiency of the enzyme phenylalanine hydroxylase, leading to failure of conversion of the essential amino-acid phenylalanine to tyrosine. Consequently, there is an accumulation of phenylalanine in the blood which if prolonged and sufficiently increased leads to brain damage. Treatment with a low phenylalanine diet prevents this. There appear to be different mutations (alleles) for phenylketonuria, so not all cases are equally severe. Those requiring drastic protein restriction are said to have the 'classical' form of the disease while others are described as 'atypical' or to have hyperphenylalaninaemia. It has become apparent over the years that the range of protein restriction needed is wide and varies considerably from child to child.

In Britain all babies are screened for phenylketonuria between the sixth and tenth day of life. The blood test, commonly known as the 'Guthrie' test is performed by the midwife usually in the baby's home. It is important that the test is done on or around the sixth day and not when the baby is born. The blood phenylalanine level will only be raised after feeding has been established and the baby has consumed some phenylalanine present in milk protein.

A blood phenylalanine level greater than 600 μmol/l with normal or low tyrosine levels is indicative of classical phenylketonuria. Normal blood levels may reach as high as 200 μmol/l. A blood level between 200 and 400 μmol/l may indicate that the child has an atypical form of phenylketonuria and further monitoring is important to assess if dietary treatment is required. It sometimes happens, particularly in breast-fed babies that blood levels are initially quite low but on transfer to diets higher in phenylalanine, for example infant formula, serum levels rise to the point where dietary restriction is indicated. For this reason, all children with blood phenylalanine levels above the normal range should be referred to a specialist centre for further evaluation. Those with classical phenylketonuria will be treated immediately, while the borderline cases will be followed carefully.

Treatment consists of a low phenylalanine diet, with a goal to maintain blood phenylalanine levels within an acceptable range (Table 11.2). Phenylalanine is present in all proteins and these need to be removed from the diet. Certain amino acids in protein are essential and must be replaced by a synthetic mixture of amino acids which does not include phenylalanine. Tyrosine, which is not normally an essential amino acid as it is synthesized from phenylalanine, becomes essential in individuals with phenylketonuria (see Fig. 11.1) and is therefore included in the amino acid supplement. The diet must be balanced in every other respect and contain adequate energy, vitamins, and minerals for growth.

In the baby this is achieved by using a specially prepared infant formula such as Lofenalac (Mead Johnson), or XP Analog (Scientific Hospital Supplies). Some of these formulas are nutritionally complete and others require additional vitamins. In the older child a special amino acid preparation such as XP Maxamaid (Scientific Hospital Supplies), Aminogran food supplement (V.C.B), and PKU 2 (Milupa) is used to provide the protein component of the diet. Some of these preparations contain carbohydrate, vitamins, and mineral whereas others require supplements. To achieve good control of plasma phenylalanine levels these amino acid preparations should be distributed evenly throughout the day.

Phenylalanine is essential for growth and must not be eliminated completely from the diet. Once the initial high phenylalanine level is reduced with the diet, phenylalanine must be reintroduced by adding either breast milk or infant formula to the diet. In the

Table 11.2. Guidelines for plasma phenylalanine concentrations in treated PKU

Age (years)	Plasma phenylalanine (μmol/l)
0–4	120–360
5–10	120–480
over 11	120–700

case of the breast-fed baby the phenylalanine free infant formula is given in a measured quantity before the baby feeds from the breast. By monitoring the blood phenylalanine level regularly the amount of breast milk and therefore phenylalanine can be controlled by increasing or decreasing the measured phenylalanine free formula. The larger the volume of phenylalanine free formula the baby is given the less breast milk he will take and the smaller the volume the more he will take. The bottle-fed baby is given a known quantity of phenylalanine as measured infant formula and then allowed to feed freely on the phenylalanine free formula.

In the older child the phenylalanine is supplied from measured portions of cereals and vegetable foods such as potato, rice, or breakfast cereals. The remaining energy requirements are met by including a variety of low phenylalanine special products (flour, biscuits, pasta), fruits, and vegetables. Many of these special products are available on prescription to patients with phenylketonuria and constitute a very important part of the diet. Care should be taken not to confuse these products with gluten free products which may contain large amounts of protein and therefore, phenylalanine.

A strict diet is recommended at least until the child reaches adolescence. After that time it may be possible to allow the blood phenylalanine levels to run within a higher range thus enabling the diet to be less strict, this still remains an area of controversy and the exact age at which the diet should be discontinued, if ever, is not clear. There is a growing body of opinion that people with phenylketonuria should be on some level of dietary restriction for life as changes in neurological functions have been seen in those who have discontinued their diet. There are, however, important difficulties associated with a lifelong diet particularly the cost of amino acid supplements. Centres are now encouraging adolescents and young adults to:

- maintain some degree of moderate protein restriction
- keep blood phenylalanine levels between 120 and 700 μmol/l
- continue to be seen for follow-up to ensure that relaxation of the diet is not causing any harm. In some areas paediatricians have established adult follow-up clinics.

A major new problem has arisen ironically as a result of the success in treating phenylketonuria. A generation of normal young women with phenylketonuria now exists. Their babies are at great risk of severe brain damage and congenital abnormality from high maternal phenylalanine levels. This damage occurs during a very early stage of embryonic development and may occur before the pregnancy is recognized. Phenylketonuric girls wishing to become pregnant must therefore follow a strict diet before conceiving and during pregnancy.

Phenylketonuria families and health professionals can receive further information and support from National Society for Phenylketonuria and Allied Disorders (see p. 246).

Organic acidaemias

The term 'organic acidaemia' is applied to any condition in which there is elevation of an abnormal organic acid in the blood. Several of these rare disorders are caused by defects in the degradation of the essential branched chain amino acids, leucine, valine, and isoleucine. The most common of these disorders are maple syrup urine disease, methylmalonic acidaemia, isovaleric acidaemia, and propionic acidaemia. The precise organic acid varies with the site of the defect.

The more severe disorders in their classical form lead to ketosis, metabolic acidosis, vomiting, and neurological abnormalities in the newborn with subsequent mental retardation if the child survives. Those less severely affected may present with recurring episodes of ketoacidosis, often precipitated by infections or a sudden increase in dietary protein and/or neurological problems, failure to thrive, or mental retardation.

The outcome for these children depends on several factors. Most important is whether the defect is due to a lack of the enzyme itself or whether it is due to a deficiency of the co-factor involved in the enzyme reaction. This in turn might be due to an abnormality of the relevant vitamin. Such vitamin dependent states or often highly responsive to mega doses of the vitamin involved. In some children where the defect is partial the residual enzyme activity is relatively high, making control easier because the child can tolerate a less restrictive diet and may not become so acutely ill.

In vitamin responsive disorders, if the diagnosis is made before irreversible damage and treatment begun sufficiently early the outlook can be excellent. Even initially poorly controlled cases may show a dramatic improvement in neurological function once the biochemical abnormality is under control.

The dietary protein restriction required varies with the severity of the disorder. In some a special amino acid supplement free from the offending branched chain amino acid is necessary. The principles of the diet are similar to those used in phenylketonuria but the exact dietary prescription must be tailored to the disorder and the individual child's requirements. In addition parents should make regular checks for urinary ketones and report immediately if these increase. Regular measurement of blood and/or urine for the specific organic acid along with other biochemical monitoring should be performed.

The major difference from phenylketonuria is the potentially devastating consequences of not adhering to the diet and the dramatic deterioration which can occur during a bout of intercurrent infection or other illness. It is important to prevent the child becoming ketoacidotic and dehydrated. The parents are therefore, advised to ensure that the child takes extra carbohydrate in the form of glucose, sugar, or glucose polymers during illness. It may be necessary to reduce the child's protein intake further and extra fluids should be encouraged. If these measures do not induce a rapid improvement the child should be admitted to hospital where intravenous glucose is given to prevent potentially fatal ketoacidosis and dehydration.

Because the child appears to be so well, parents can be lulled into a false sense of security. It is very important that they do not relax their vigilance or be tempted into thinking that the child is 'cured' and no longer at risk of an acute crisis.

Galactosaemia

Galactose appears in the urine in three specific inborn errors of metabolism:

- classical galactosaemia
- galactokinase deficiency
- epimerase deficiency

Classical galactosaemia

Galactosaemia is an autosomal recessive inherited disorder. The basic defect is a deficiency of galactose-1-phosphate uridyl-transferase which is necessary to metabolize galactose to glucose phosphate. The incidence of classical galactosaemia is approximately 1:44 000 births.

The presentation depends on the severity of the disorder. Some infants die unexpectedly before the diagnosis is made. Less acute cases may have persisting neonatal jaundice with vomiting, diarrhoea, and impaired liver function with hepatomegaly. Some infants are referred because they are failing to thrive. Cataract may be present at an early stage.

Biochemical findings include a raised galactose-1-phosphate in erythrocytes and low or absent transferase activity in whole blood. Initially the condition must be treated as a medical emergency because sudden death from hypoglycaemia is not unusual.

When a reducing substance other than glucose is found in the urine the infant is started on a galactose-free diet immediately. This will lead to a rapid improvement and a reduction in the galactose-1-phosphate levels. The diet should be continued for life. With early diagnosis and strict dietary compliance one would expect a good outlook. Unfortunately, for some as yet unknown reason, the long-term prognosis is not as good as for phenyl-ketonuria. Some children develop complications of mental disability, speech defects, ovarian failure, and neurological syndromes despite complying with diet. There is need for further research to consider the levels of dietary restriction necessary and to determine other factors which may influence outcome, but endogenous synthesis of galactose is one recently recognized factor.

A galactose-free diet requires the exclusion of all galactose containing foods. Galactose is a monosaccharide found as a component of the disaccharide lactose. It is therefore, necessary to exclude all lactose from the diet which in effect means following a milk-free diet. Care should also be taken to avoid other food and non-food items such as drugs which may contain lactose.

A soya formula such as Wysoy (SMA Nutrition), InfaSoy (Cow & Gate, Nutricia), or a special preparation such as Galactomin 17 (Cow and Gate, Nutricia) should be used. The exclusion of galactosides, found in many vegetables and legumes, from the diet is an area of current debate. However in the UK, opinion favours the continued inclusion of these foods and dietary limitations are not required.

Children with galactosaemia should be followed regularly with monitoring of red blood cell galactose-1-phosphate levels and dietary review. It is important to arrange for psychological testing to be carried out from time to time.

Galactokinase and epimerase deficiency

Galactokinase deficiency is due to a defect of the enzyme galactokinase and leads to accumulation of galactose in the lens of the eye causing cataracts. There is no effect on neurodevelopment. Treatment requires galactose avoidance. Epimerase deficiency is an extremely rare condition and has a very poor prognosis.

Glycogen storage disease

Another group of disorders of carbohydrate metabolism are those of glycogen storage. These include glycogen storage disease (GSD) types I, II, and III and the phosphorylase system deficiencies. In all forms of GSD careful monitoring of growth and nutritional requirements is necessary and these children should be followed in a specialist centre.

Glycogen storage disease type I (GSDI)

In this form of GSD there is either a deficiency of glucose-6-phosphatase or a defect in one of its transport proteins. Clinical manifestations include growth retardation and hepatomegaly. The main goal of dietary treatment is to promote normal growth by maintaining a normal blood glucose level and this requires frequent administration of dietary glucose throughout the 24-hour period. This generally necessitates frequent carbohydrate-containing meals and snacks during the day, often including drinks of a glucose polymer or uncooked cornstarch preparations (for slower glucose release). Overnight nasogastric feeding is used to provide glucose while the child is asleep.

Glycogen storage disease type II

This form of GSD is caused by a deficiency of acid maltase, leading to an accumulation of glycogen. The infantile form (Pompe's disease) is associated with a poor prognosis and early death. The childhood form is less severe presenting with generalized muscle weakness which may lead to cardio-respiratory insufficiency and death. Dietary treatment includes a high protein diet with decreased intakes of carbohydrate and fat to provide normal energy intake.

Glycogen storage disease type III

GSDIII involves a deficiency of the glycogen debranching enzyme and the production of glucose from glycogen is limited. Hypoglycaemia and poor growth are common in childhood but symptoms become less severe as the child gets older. Dietary management varies according to the severity of the disease but includes a high protein diet. Some children also require frequent feeding similar to that used for GSD type I and overnight feedings may be used.

Disorders of the phosphorylase system

These have similar symptoms to GSDIII, but are much milder with minimal hypoglycaemia. Adults are usually asymptomatic and there is a normal life expectancy.

Diabetes mellitus

Diabetes mellitus in children requires insulin and symptoms cannot be treated using tablets as with some forms of maturity onset diabetes mellitus. The classical symptoms of juvenile diabetes mellitus are acute onset polyuria, polydipsia, weight loss, raised blood sugar, and glycosuria. The treatment of insulin injections and diet aim to normalize blood glucose levels enabling the child to lead a fully active normal life.

The child should be referred immediately to the local paediatric diabetic team so that treatment can be commenced. In most areas, the child will be admitted to hospital for a few days and management continued at home with the support of outreach services. The aim of initial treatment is to normalize the blood glucose level by giving appropriate insulin injections along with a suitable diet. During this time the child and family are taught the basics of treatment. This includes testing blood glucose, insulin injections, recognition of different insulins, drawing up the correct dose, injection technique, rotation of injection sites, and care of syringe and needles. They are also taught the basic principles of diet modification and how to deal with various emergency situations.

Further teaching includes dealing with hypoglycaemia, the need for extra carbohydrate during exercise, going on holiday, and other problems of daily life as they occur. These and other refinements of treatment can be learned over a longer period of time.

The dietary treatment for the diabetic child aims to provide:

• a nutritionally balanced diet, incorporating healthy eating practices
• adequate nutrition for optimal growth.

When the child is first seen by the dietitian, a dietary history will be taken and the dietary prescription made taking into account the individual child's nutritional requirements. The nutritional requirements of diabetic children are much the same as other normal healthy children. Dietary recommendations include:

• carbohydrates to provide a minimum of 40 % energy intake, usually around 50 % energy in children over 5 years; the formula 120 g + 10 g for every year of life meets this recommendation
• fibre intake should be 2 g/100 kcal/day, starting at 1 g/100 kcal/day in children who are used to much lower intakes and gradually increasing

- fat intake should provide no more than 35 % energy in children over 5 years of age
- protein intake should meet normal requirements
- adequate energy to meet requirements according to age, size, and activity levels.

The diet is normally based on a carbohydrate exchange system and the children are advised to divide the daily carbohydrate allowance between three meals and three snacks according to the child's usual meal pattern and the type of insulin. This initial carbohydrate prescription usually requires modification within the first few weeks, often after the child has regained any weight lost.

The carbohydrates are divided into 10 gram exchanges. One carbohydrate exchange when eaten in a specified amount contains 10 grams of carbohydrate (Table 11.3). The British Diabetic Association produces a list of standard carbohydrate exchanges and information regarding the carbohydrate content of manufactured foods. It is important that other foods are also included in the diet and that healthy food choices are made. In some centres an unmeasured diet is used; however, regular meals and snacks

Table 11.3. Some examples of 10 g carbohydrate exchanges

Wholemeal bread	1 small slice
White bread	1 small slice
Weetabix	1 biscuit
All Bran, Bran Flakes	5 tablespoons
Porridge	7 tablespoons
Cornflakes	5 tablespoons
Crackers	2
Digestive biscuit	1 biscuit
Boiled potato	1 small
Mashed potato	1 scoop
Apple	1
Orange	1
Banana	1
Milk; semi-skimmed, whole, skimmed	⅓ pint (1 glass)
Fruit sweetened yoghurt	½ carton

are still important and an emphasis is placed upon healthy food choices including high-fibre carbohydrate foods.

Families with a diabetic child are advised to join the British Diabetic Association and children are encouraged to participate in the diabetic camps organized by the association. The camps are supervised by trained staff including doctors, nurses, and dietitians and provide the diabetic child with the chance to meet others with the same condition and to learn how they cope with their diabetes. The children are encouraged to participate in a wide range of activities and are taught about self-care and control of their condition.

Ketogenic diet for epilepsy

The ketogenic diet was first used as a treatment for epilepsy in the 1920s, since then it has gone through various stages of popularity but has not been rigorously evaluated. It appears to be most successful in the treatment of myoclonic, focal, and temporal lobe epilepsy, but is often used as the last resort where drug treatments have failed. In recent years there has been some renewed interest in the treatment of epilepsy with a ketogenic diet, especially in the more traditional diet based on normal high fat foods. The object of the diet is to induce a level of ketosis by giving a very low carbohydrate, high fat diet. The diet is very difficult to follow and requires careful medical and nutritional monitoring in a centre experienced in planning these diets. Initiation of the diet requires hospitalization with a brief period of starvation before the diet is introduced. The classical ketogenic diet usually consists of 4 g of fat to every 1 g of protein and carbohydrate. This high fat diet is achieved by using large quantities of foods such as double cream and butter, it is very restrictive and requires detailed calculations to ensure adequate nutrition. The diet is usually recommended for a minimum period of 3 months and may be continued for up to 3 years. It does cause some degree of growth retardation which is often compensated for after the diet is discontinued. The diet is stopped gradually by reintroducing a more normal carbohydrate and protein intake.

over a 5–10 days period. In those children where the diet is successful, improvement continues after the diet ceases.

Selected references

Freeman, J.M., Kelly, M.T., and Freeman, J.B. (1996, second ed.). *The epilepsy diet treatment, an introduction to the ketogenic diet.* Demos, New York, USA.

MacDonald, A. (1996). Nutritional management of cystic fibrosis. *Archives of Disease in Childhood*, **74**, 81–7.

MacDonald, A., Rylance, G., Hall, S.K., Asplin, D., and Booth, I.W. (1996). Factors affecting the variation in plasma phenylalanine in patients with phenylketonuria on diet. *Archives of Disease in Childhood*, **74**, 412–17.

Nutrition Subcommittee of the Professional Advisory Committee of the British Diabetic Association. (1989). Dietary recommendations for children and adolescents with diabetes. *Diabetic Medicine*, **6**, 537–47.

Peckham, D., Leonard, C., Range, S., and Knox, A. (1996). Nutritional status and pulmonary function in patients with cystic fibrosis and without Burkholderia cepacia colonization: role of specialist dietetic support. *J. Hum. Nutr. Dietet*, **9**, 173–9.

Segal, S. (1995). Galactosaemia unsolved. *European Journal of Pediatrics*, **154**, (7), (supplement 2), 97–102.

....

12

Nutritional management in chronic disease

In recent years it has become established clinical practice to try to reverse the malnutrition associated with chronic conditions such as inflammatory bowel disease, cystic fibrosis, heart disease, and AIDS. Studies of children in hospital with chronic illness have indicated a surprisingly high prevalence of malnutrition (in the order of 30%), and this has often gone unrecognized. Although evidence for the value of nutritional intervention in terms of altering the natural history of disease has not been unequivocally demonstrated in all of these conditions, many clinicians regard nutritional restitution as being of undoubted benefit to the patient. This is because protein-energy malnutrition not only leads to growth failure, but has potentially serious consequences for all systems of the body:

- gastrointestinal tract   -hypochlorhydria
                                  -reduced mucosal function
                                  -pancreatic exocrine insufficiency
- immune system   -impaired cell mediated immunity
- respiratory system   -reduced inspiratory force
- cardio-vascular   -myocardial dysfunction

- musculo-skeletal   -muscle wasting
- central nervous system -apathy; depression
                                     -possible delay in intellectual
                                     development

Taking these considerations into account, together with evidence that malnutrition may be associated with an increased risk of morbidity and mortality following surgical procedures, has given impetus to the search for methods of providing optimal nutritional care.

Enteral tube feeding

In many cases where an individual child is unable to maintain an adequate voluntary intake of food, effective nutritional support can be given using specialized liquid feeds delivered by accurate and portable enteral feeding pumps via nasogastric or gastrostomy tubes (see Fig. 12.1). These may be given as sole nutritional support, or as a supplement to normal diet.

It is difficult to give precise guidance as to when tube feeding should be given to children with chronic disorders, but the conditions that are usually fulfilled before starting enteral nutritional support are shown in Table 12.1.

Parenteral feeding

Parenteral feeding (sometimes confusingly referred to as 'hyperalimentation') is the delivery of nutrients directly into the blood via an intravenous catheter, thus bypassing the bowel. It is most commonly given for relatively short periods of time to children with temporary 'gut failure' precluding enteral feeding. Only in rare instances is long-term parenteral nutrition a necessary alternative to enteral nutrition. If the gastrointestinal tract is functional it is desirable to give enteral rather than parenteral feeding as it is associated with fewer complications and is more simple to manage. It is often said that another advantage of enteral

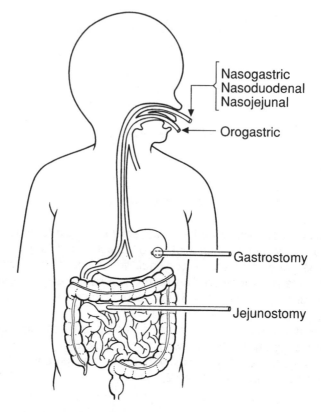

Fig. 12.1. Accessing the gut during enteral nutritional support.

feeding is lower cost; however, in the context of the overall cost of intensive care (where the 'enteral or parenteral?' debate usually takes place), this is probably not an important consideration. The indications for parenteral nutrition are shown in Table 12.2.

Home nutritional support

Both enteral tube feeding and parenteral nutrition can be managed at home with the aid of community services and/or commercial home care companies. This is an expanding area of

Table 12.1. Indications for starting enteral nutritional support in chronically-ill children

Impaired energy intake	• usually 50–60% of EAR despite high energy supplements
together with	
Severe and deteriorating wasting	• weight for height > 2 standard deviations below the mean • skinfold thickness < third centile
and/or	
Depressed linear growth	• fall in height of > 0.3 standard deviations per year
or	
	• height velocity < 5 cm per year
or	
	• decrease in height velocity of at least 2 cm from the preceding year during early to mid puberty

Table 12.2. Indications for parenteral nutrition

Newborn	
Absolute indications	intestinal failure (short bowel, functional immaturity, pseudo-obstruction) necrotizing enterocolitis
Relative indications	respiratory distress promotion of growth in preterm infants possible prevention of necrotizing enterocolitis
Older infants and children	
Intestinal failure	short bowel protracted diarrhoea chronic intestinal pseudo-obstruction post-operative abdominal or cardio-thoracic surgery radiation/cytotoxic therapy
Exclusion of luminal nutrients	Crohn's disease pancreatitis
Organ failure	acute renal failure acute liver failure
Hyper-catabolism	extensive burns severe trauma

clinical care in the UK although still bedevilled by confusion and argument over funding arrangements. It is to be hoped that in the future, purchasing authorities will develop specific contracts with provider units for home care, including home nutritional support. The British Association for Parenteral and Enteral Nutrition (BAPEN) representing both patients and professionals, has produced guidelines for good practice in relation both to home enteral and parenteral nutrition.

The conditions associated with failure to thrive and for which home enteral tube feeding (HETF) may be used include:

- neurological disorders (e.g. cerebral palsy, head injury, degenerative central nervous system disease)
- gastro-oesophageal reflux
- cystic fibrosis
- liver disease
- chronic renal failure
- heart disease
- malignancy
- short bowel syndrome
- Crohn's disease

A clinical nurse specialist in nutrition (CNSN) working together with paediatrician, surgeon, dietitian, and pharmacist as part of a multidisciplinary nutritional care team plays a key role in preparing children and their families for home nutritional support prior to discharge from hospital, as well as coordinating support and follow-up after they return home. Responses to HETF are generally very positive and many families consider the advantages far outweigh the disadvantages.

An improvement in the overall state of well-being of children on HETF is seen as one of the major benefits, together with a sense of freedom from having to struggle unsuccessfully with achieving nutritional goals from table food and supplementary drinks. Negative aspects include distress with passage of nasogastric tubes, and the inevitable unwelcome attention these draw from other people. We believe that this is one of the reasons for choosing gastrostomy feeding if it is anticipated that nutritional support is likely to be required for more than three months, with the exception of some children with liver disease. Follow-up studies of children receiving home enteral nutrition have demonstrated that it is effective in improving nutritional status for a variety of different indications, although the benefits are short lived in some cases when feeding is discontinued.

Gastrostomy feeding

Although insertion of a gastrostomy used to be performed as an open surgical procedure, it is now much more common for insertion to be carried out using a percutaneous endoscopic technique. In children who require anti-reflux surgery as well as a gastrostomy, an operative approach is still used. Prior to insertion parents and children are seen on a number of occasions by the CNSN who demonstrates the gastrostomy device and makes plans for discharge home. Careful nutritional assessment by the team allows goals to be set and the appropriate feed to be selected to meet the nutritional needs of the individual child. After gastrostomy insertion, the CNSN:

- teaches care of the gastrostomy and safe delivery of feed
- contacts health support staff in the community
- arranges continuing support for the family (including home and school visits)
- arranges supply of equipment

When the gastrostomy tube has been in place for six weeks we generally replace it with a low profile device (the MIC-key, Ballard Medical Products). These are unobtrusive (Fig. 12.2), reliable, well tolerated by children, and liked by their parents.

The CNSN is used as the first point of contact when there are any problems with the gastrostomy at home. She can assist in resolution of these problems drawing on the expertise of other team members when necessary. Difficulties most commonly encountered are:

- a faulty valve allowing leakage of gastric fluid
- wound granulation around the insertion site
- burst intra-gastric balloon
- accidental removal

**Balloon Inflation
Valve**

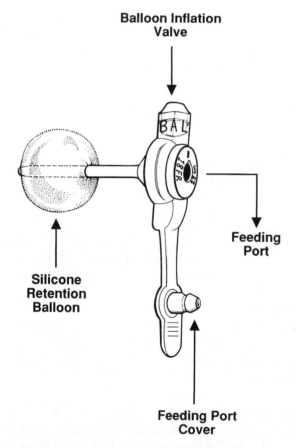

**Feeding
Port**

**Silicone
Retention
Balloon**

**Feeding Port
Cover**

Fig. 12.2. Low profile 'button' gastrostomy device.

These complications are relatively infrequent and usually easy to deal with.

Children receiving HETF should be carefully monitored and regular contact with paediatrician, nurse, and dietitian will be required. In order to meet the constantly changing nutritional needs of the growing and developing child, it is important period- ically, to adjust the volume and type of feed being given.

Feeding pumps

Enteral feeding pumps are used to administer liquid tube feeds by continuous infusion, particularly at night time. Parents and older children need to be taught how to use the pump, which ideally should be simple to operate, accurate, quiet, portable, and have inbuilt safety alarms indicating disconnection, blockage, or running out of feed. Few combine all these features and we currently prefer to use a pump which will operate on mains or batteries such as the 'Kangaroo 2100' or the Abbott 'Flexiflo Companion'. A portable pump such as these with its own carrying pack can be used for children who require continuous feeds and attend school during the day. An unobtrusive carrying pack for a pump and litre of feed can be improvized from a sports bag or small backpack (Fig. 12.3), or obtained from the pump manufacturer.

Feeds used for HETF

Age, size, and gastrointestinal function will dictate the choice of feed. An infant with normal digestive function requiring HETF can be fed either expressed breast milk or infant formula with additives to increase the calorie content as necessary. The toddler and older child can be given one of the special paediatric formulas listed in Table 12.3. A modified paediatric formula is usually used for children over five years of age. Adult formulae can be used in older children and adolescents but may require modification.

Sometimes a special formula may be required for particular diseases or when there is impaired gastrointestinal function. We have considered the use of some of these in the sections on liver and inflammatory bowel disease; however, detailed discussion is beyond the scope of this book.

Complications of home enteral nutrition

In our experience serious complications of home enteral tube feeding are extremely rare, although major aspiration, entanglement in tubing, and enterocutaneous fistula have been reported in the literature. However, some minor problems are relatively

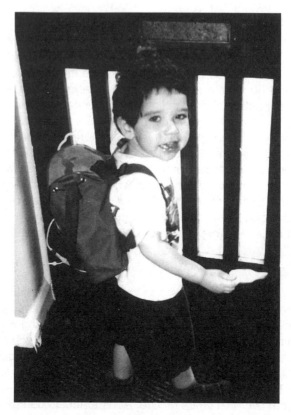

Fig. 12.3. Carrying pack for enteral feeding pump.

Table 12.3. Some complete formulas used in enteral feeding

Infant	Children aged 1–5 years
Expressed breast milk	Paediasure
Cow's milk based infant formula	(*Ross Laboratories*)
Soya based infant formula	Nutrison Paediatric Standard
	Nutrison Paediatric Energy Plus
	(*Cow & Gate Nutricia*)
	Frebini
	(*Fresenius*)

common. For example sleep is often disturbed with parents getting up to check volume of feed delivered, or by pump alarms sounding. Children may wake more often because of nocturia, or the need to open their bowels in the night. The majority of families seem able to take such problems in their stride. Prolonged tube feeding sometimes results in reluctance to take food by mouth at a later stage, particularly in the young infant. The risk of this potentially serious complication can be minimized by continuing to offer oral stimulation and some food by mouth whenever possible. The early involvement of a speech therapist who specializes in feeding problems can be invaluable in helping to avoid such problems.

Home parenteral nutrition

Home Parenteral Nutrition (HPN) allows children with long-term expectation of dependency on intravenous feeding to be cared for at home. The usual indications are chronic intestinal failure as a result of short bowel syndrome, intractable diarrhoea with malabsorption, or severe abnormalities of gut motility. Unlike North America and parts of Europe, HPN is still relatively uncommon in the UK where perhaps no more than 40–50 children at any one time are managed in this way. It is likely that overall costs of care are far less in the community than in hospital (currently estimated as £25 000 and £100 000 per annum respectively), and this has often been the main driving force behind developments in other countries. Although a major undertaking for families, HPN does offer children who would otherwise be institutionalized, a good quality of life, the possibility of fully realising growth and developmental potential, and a reduced risk of some parenteral nutrition related complications such as central venous catheter sepsis. Most can attend school and take part in normal social life including sporting activities and holidays.

Before HPN can be considered, children need to be stable from the point of view of their medical condition, and parents or caregivers have to have considerable motivation as well as suitable accommodation. An intensive training programme together with an ongoing support service is necessary for families, and, as in home enteral feeding, the role of the CNSN is crucial. Provision of written information relating to equipment, procedures and problem solving is essential for caregivers, who should also be given their own folder including an up to date summary of their child's medical problems to show to unfamiliar medical and nursing staff when the need arises. Supply of equipment is usually arranged through one of the commercial home care companies. An entire room at home may need to be given over to storage space for disposables including two weeks worth of refrigerated PN fluids. Disposal of sharps and clinical waste has to be arranged with the local authority and the electricity company needs to be informed of the importance of maintaining supply.

Feeds are delivered via a central venous catheter and usually given overnight. The catheter is then disconnected and closed off during the day allowing the child mobility and freedom from infusion equipment. Unfortunately, major thromboembolic events (pulmonary emboli) are now recognized as a major life-threatening complication of prolonged PN. Studies are in progress to determine ways in which this complication might be prevented. Small bowel transplantation as an alternative to long-term PN in gastrointestinal failure is only just advancing beyond the experimental phase, but in time is likely to become an option for some children.

Specific disorders commonly requiring nutritional intervention

The rest of this chapter covers some of the specific diseases where nutrition is an integral component of treatment.

Liver disease

Protein-energy malnutrition affects over 60% of children with severe liver disease and has an adverse affect on the outcome of liver transplantation. Anorexia and fat maldigestion are important contributory factors, particularly in the child with cholestasis. Liver disease (Fig. 12.4) is often associated with fluid retention

Facial telangiectasia

Spider naevi

Splenomegaly

Hepatomegaly

Jaundice

Large abdomen

Vasodilation

↑ Cardiac output

↑ Aldosterone

Ascites

Oedema

↓ Muscle bulk

↓ Skinfold thickness

Cutaneous shunts

Clubbing

Palmar erythema

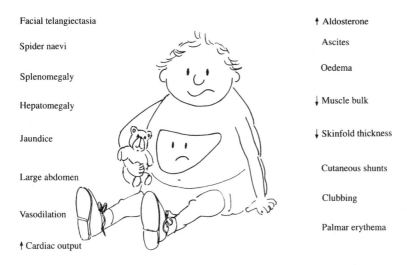

Fig. 12.4. Liver disease in children. (reproduced by kind permission Nom Ball).

which means that weight measurements are misleading. A full anthropometric assessment should be performed if nutritional status is to be assessed accurately. Mid-arm circumference and triceps skinfold thickness less than the teath centile are pointers to the need for nutritional intervention.

Depending on the severity of liver disease, energy intake may need to be increased to 140–200% of the estimated average requirement. This large increase in energy needs is due to an increase in resting energy requirement and, in some cases, fat malabsorption due to a reduction or loss of bile salt production and bile flow. The exact nutritional needs will vary with each individual child but modifications in the type and amount of fat in the diet or feed is often required. Special supplements such as glucose polymer, or medium chain triglycerides (MCT) can be used to increase the energy content of the diet. A gradual increase is usually required to prevent complications of diarrhoea caused by the increased osmolality of feeds containing these supplements.

Protein requirements may also be increased, and intake can go up to 4 g/kg/day without precipitating hepatic encephalopathy. The risks of essential fatty acid and fat soluble vitamin deficiencies are increased. The precise requirements for essential fatty acids are unknown, but large doses of fat soluble vitamins may be necessary (e.g. 5000–20000 units of vitamin A, 100–800 mg vitamin E, 50–150 µg/kg of alphacalcidol, and 5–10 mg vitamin K daily).

The anorexia experienced by most children with severe liver disease means that tube feeding is commonly required if nutritional goals are to be met. A nasogastric tube is preferable to gastrostomy in these patients because of complications related to ascites and the future need for abdominal access during liver transplantation.

In summary, the following considerations make nutritional support necessary in liver disease:

- increased resting energy requirements
- anorexia
- fat malabsorption
- disturbed metabolism
- adverse affects of malnutrition on prognosis.

Inflammatory bowel disease

Ulcerative colitis and Crohn's disease are both chronic inflammatory conditions of unknown cause which affect the bowel, and for which there is no specific curative treatment. Whilst Crohn's disease most commonly involves the terminal ileum and colon, any part of the gastrointestinal tract from mouth to anus may be affected. Ulcerative colitis is confined to the large bowel. Recent epidemiological studies suggest that the incidence of Crohn's disease is on the increase affecting around 3 per 10000 children; ulcerative colitis is about one third as common and does not appear to be increasing in frequency.

Growth failure and malnutrition are common complications of inflammatory bowel disease, and seen in 5–10% of children with ulcerative colitis and perhaps as many as 30% of those with Crohn's disease. Important factors include anorexia, increased nutrient utilization and requirements, abnormal losses from the gastrointestinal tract, drug treatment, surgery, and malabsorption. Nutritional support should be regarded very much as part of the management of these conditions, with steroids and anti-inflammatory medications being the main medical interventions. Restitution of nutritional status can be achieved through provision of a balanced diet supplemented with high protein, high calorie formulas, or in some cases with liquid formula alone.

Dietary intervention in Crohn's disease may be used as a primary therapy to reduce inflammation. A liquid diet, usually in the form of an elemental feed such as Elemental 028 (Scientific Hospital Supplies) may be used to induce a remission of disease activity, and has been shown to be as effective as steroid treatment. A number of suggestions have been advanced to explain this anti-inflammatory effect of elemental diet:

- reduction of antigenic effect of food proteins
- changes in intestinal microflora
- reduction of secretory abnormalities of the bowel mucosa
- improvement of intestinal permeability
- possible improvement in disordered immunological function.

The feed is usually given for a period of six weeks, with exclusion of all other food and drinks (except water). Single foods are then reintroduced over several weeks as the volume of elemental feed is reduced. Such liquid feeds are unpalatable and nasogastric tube feeding is usually preferred. When repeated episodes of elemental diet are required, or if a nasogastric tube is refused, a gastrostomy should be considered. Recently a polymeric liquid feed containing whole protein (Nutrison Standard, Nutricia) has also been shown capable of inducing remission, and has the advantage of greater palatability. Other whole protein formulas may also have this effect. Although elemental diets were thought to be most beneficial in children with small bowel disease, it is now clear that some children with Crohn's disease affecting the colon also respond to this form of dietary management.

Renal disease

Nutritional problems loom large in the management of children with chronic renal disease particularly those who are in chronic renal failure.

There are also many children with chronic renal conditions which will never cause renal failure or who will remain with relatively good renal function for many years. Some conditions do not cause renal failure in themselves but may predispose to hypertension in later life. Good dietary care by an experienced paediatric dietitian, as part of the multidisciplinary renal team is essential to the proper management of children with chronic renal disease and is a principle reason why all such children should attend a paediatric nephrology clinic.

Chronic renal failure

Chronic renal failure (CRF) is often associated with poor growth and malnutrition and dietary intervention is an important component of care. Children with CRF have major nutritional problems both before dialysis and transplantation and after the need for such management becomes imperative. As with other aspects of management, ideally diet and the changes it will undergo during different phases of the process should be seen by the child and its family as a logical progression, so that they will not be faced with sudden, unwelcome and unpleasant dietary alterations.

It is essential to ensure that the parents and the child understand how important it is that the child should grow as normally as possible and this is linked to adequate intakes of nutrients and energy. For several reasons, some related to the underlying disease causing the renal failure, some due to the effects of renal failure itself and also because of important psychological factors, children with renal failure are often anorexic, eat poorly, and as a consequence suffer from malnutrition, poor linear growth, and weight gain. It may be possible, by ensuring that nutrition forms an integral part of multidisciplinary management, to prevent or lessen these difficulties.

As in many chronic conditions children with renal failure are faddy and have their own ideas about what they will or will not eat. They are likely to use food as a weapon in the eternal battle with adults and be determined to want what is considered 'unhealthy' and to reject what is regarded as good. The principle of success lies in gaining the confidence of the parents and providing additional support through family therapy and support groups to anticipate and prevent eating disorders and related growth problems.

The approach we use is to find out what the child finds acceptable and to attempt to build up energy and nutrient intake around this. The diet should be based on usual family eating patterns. If the household is one in which there is little food preparation or cooking then it will be based on suitable processed foods supplemented as necessary.

In some children eating becomes such a battle and intake so poor that gastrostomy tube feeding should be considered. This can take the pressure away from eating and allow the child to enjoy small amounts of food at family mealtimes whilst nutrition is taken care of by an overnight gastrostomy feed.

Dietary treatment for CRF will vary according to the state of the disease and the form of treatment. There are generally three stages of treatment for CRF:

• pre-dialysis
• peritoneal or haemodialysis
• transplantation

Before dialysis becomes necessary the aims of nutritional intervention are to:

• maintain normal growth
• prevent nausea and vomiting by controlling uraemia
• slow the progression of deteriorating renal function
• maintain as normal a life-style as possible

Provision of adequate energy intake is essential and usually requires energy supplements such as glucose polymers or Duocal (Scientific hospital supplies) (glucose polymer and fat which provides more calories). Some degree of protein restriction is often necessary to control uraemia and hyperphosphataemia; however, low protein diets do run the risk of contributing to malnutrition.

In all stages of treatment the dietary goals are:

- to promote normal growth through adequate energy intake
- regulate protein intake according to growth needs and type of treatment
- balance fluid and electrolytes
- regulate calcium and phosphate intake to promote normal bone growth
- provide adequate intake of all vitamins and minerals

Once the child is on dialysis the diet is tailored to the type of treatment and the individual child's requirements. For example on peritoneal dialysis a high protein diet is necessary, whereas on haemodialysis a lower protein intake is appropriate.

In addition to the multivitamin supplement usually given, vitamin D either as calcitriol or alpha-calcidol should be prescribed once the blood creatinine is clearly elevated with the hope of minimizing metabolic bone disease.

The best index of successful nutritional management is growth and so it is essential that a good record be kept of height and weight measurements which should be plotted on a centile chart.

Nephrotic syndrome

The main nutritional problems in children with minimal change nephrotic syndrome (MCNS) who require repeated steroid treatment are obesity and growth failure. Most children with nephrotic syndrome have so called MCNS. This is more common in boys and usually affects preschoolchildren. The cause of MCNS is not known, but most respond well to corticosteroid treatment and require little dietary intervention. Children vary in the degree to which they become overweight with steroid treatment. The appetite is often greatly increased and in those with a predisposition to obesity quite alarming weight gain may ensue which in a few individuals does not revert on cessation of treatment. It may be wise if there is a family history of obesity of begin calorie restriction with the beginning of treatment rather than to wait until obesity has actually manifested itself.

Nutritional management involves:

- a balanced diet with adequate energy and protein intake to promote normal growth and prevent wasting
- monitor energy intake and weight gain to avoid obesity
- no added salt diet to help reduce thirst and oedema
- some fluid restriction may be necessary in initial oedematous phase
- a healthy diet avoiding excess fat and saturated fat, especially important for the child who is resistant to steroid treatment

Human immunodeficiency virus infection

The acquired immune deficiency syndrome (AIDS) is due to infection with a retrovirus, the human immunodeficiency virus (HIV). AIDS is now a major health problem throughout the world, with a predicted prevalence of 150 million infected people world-wide by the year 2005. HIV-infected individuals eventually develop immunodeficiency predominantly as a result of depletion in the number of CD4 positive 'helper' T-cells leading to failure to mount specific immune responses to antigens. The individual then becomes susceptible to opportunistic infections, particularly those caused by viruses, protozoa, and fungi. In addition, susceptibility to malignancies such as lymphoma and Kaposi's sarcoma is greatly increased.

Between 15 and 30 % of children born to HIV-positive mothers are themselves infected. Diagnosis is based on a clinical picture of AIDS, the presence of virus or antigen, or the presence of HIV antibodies after 18 months of age. Of those children who are HIV-infected, about one third develop serious HIV symptoms or AIDS in the first year of life. Some children do not develop symptoms until 4–6 years of age, and may not develop AIDS until adolescence. Growth failure has been reported in 25–100 % of children with symptomatic HIV infection and has been associated with significantly shortened survival time. Infection, malignancy and treatments can all result in weight loss through a combination of factors including poor appetite, diarrhoea, malabsorption, nausea, vomiting, and lethargy. Poor growth may be an even earlier indication of HIV infection than the decline in CD4 lymphocyte count and the development of opportunistic infection.

Maintaining good nutrition is an important part of general supportive care, which together with therapy and prophylaxis of opportunistic infection and antiretroviral treatment can contribute to quality of life and life expectancy. Breast-feeding is a route of transmission of HIV infection to the newborn and doubles the risk of infant infection. The virus is found in cells within breast milk in the majority of HIV infected women. In developed countries bottle-feeding is advocated, whereas in less developed countries the risks of not breast-feeding have to be balanced against the risks of breast-feeding. Immunosuppression in advanced HIV disease, and vitamin A deficiency appear to increase the risk of mother-infant transmission.

There is relatively little information regarding the safety and efficacy of aggressive nutritional intervention in symptomatic children. Tube feeding has been shown to improve weight gain but not to improve linear growth or muscle mass. This may be because some children have an increased resting energy expenditure, or have endocrine abnormalities as part of the multisystem disorder caused by HIV infection. In children with chronic diarrhoea and malabsorption, parenteral feeding is a possible alternative to enteral nutritional support, but requires careful consideration as to whether or not this is really in the best interests of the child. Children with HIV infection (particularly those with diarrhoea) are at risk of micronutrient deficiencies including folate, zinc, iron, and selenium.

Nutritional care for the child who is infected with HIV or has AIDS requires due consideration and dietary intervention will depend on the child's needs. These will vary as the disease progresses and with phases of treatment. In general, vitamin and mineral supplementation to normal RNI levels is needed, together with other dietary supplements as necessary. Greater understanding of these children's unique needs will undoubtedly develop as new insights are gained from research.

Cancer

There are three main types of cancers seen in children:

- leukaemias
- lymphomas
- solid tumours

Malnutrition is a common problem in children with cancer and to a large extent is caused by the treatment and its complications. Normal eating fads also play a role in the development of malnutrition along with other psychological factors.

Detailed nutritional assessment is essential in the diagnosis of malnutrition and alternatives to the more usual height and weight measurements (see Chapter 1) may be required because large tumour masses can distort body weight.

Nutritional support for children with cancer will depend on:

- the degree of malnutrition
- the side effects of treatment which may affect eating, e.g. nausea and vomiting, diarrhoea, sore mouth, taste changes
- the nutritional needs of the individual child.

In some children additional dietary supplements will help provide a nutritionally adequate diet, in others nutritional support in the form of tube feedings or occasionally parenteral nutrition may be required. Current research suggests that tolerance to chemotherapy and outcome are improved with improved nutritional status.

Alternative diets or fad diets are often claimed to be a cure for cancer, these diets can pose a serious health risk to children and are not recommended. If parents wish to pursue such a diet they should seek dietetic advice to modify the diet so that is provides adequate nutrition for the growing child.

Further reading

Grunow, J.E., Chait, P., Savoie, S., Mullan, C., and Pencharz, P. (1994). Gastrostomy feeding. In *Recent advances in paediatrics* (ed. T.J. David), pp. 23–39. Churchill Livingstone, London.

Holden, C.E., Puntis, J.W.L., Charlton, C.P.L., and Booth, I.W. (1991). Nasogastric feeding at home: acceptability and safety. *Archives of Disease in Childhood*, **66**, 148–51.

Kleinman, R.E., Balistreri, W.F., Heyman, M.B., Kirschner, B.S., Lake, A.M., Motil, K.J., Seidman, E., and Udall, J.N. (1989). Nutritional support for pediatric patients with inflammatory bowel disease. *Journal of Pediatric Gastroenterology and Nutrition*, **8**, 8–12.

Macallan, D.C. and Griffin, G.E. (1995). Nutrition support in human immunodeficiency virus infection. In *Artifical nutrition support in clinical practice*, (ed. J. Payne-James, G. Grimble, and D. Silk), pp. 493–509. Edward Arnold, London.

Norman, L.J., Coleman, J.E., and Watson, A.R. (1995). Nutritional management in a child on chronic peritoneal dialysis: a team approach. *Journal of Human Nutrition and Dietetics*, 8, 209–13.

Report of a working party chaired by Professor J.E. Lennard-Jones (1992). *A positive approach to nutrition as treatment*. King's Fund Centre, London.

Further reading and references

Belton, N.R. and Williams, A.F. (ed.) (1991). *Textbook of paediatric nutrition*, McLaren, D.S. and Burman, D., Churchill Livingstone, London.

British National Formulary (1996). British Medical Association and The Pharmaceutical Society of Great Britain.

Cooper, P.J. and Stein, A. (ed.) (1992). *Feeding problems and eating disorders in children and adolescents*. Harwood Academic Publishers, Reading.

Department of Health and Social Security (1988). *Present day practice in infant feeding*. Report on Health and Social Subjects Number 32. HMSO, London.

Department of Health, (1989). *The diets of British schoolchildren*. Report on Health and Social Subjects Number 36. HMSO, London.

Department of Health, (1991). *Dietary reference values for food energy and nutrients for the United Kingdom*. Report on Health and Social Subjects Number 41. HMSO, London.

Department of Health, (1995). *Weaning and the weaning diet*. Report on Health and Social Subject Number 45. HMSO, London.

Department of Health, (1994). *Nutritional aspects of cardiovascular disease*. Report on Health and Social Subjects Number 46. HMSO, London.

Henschel, D. and Inch, S. (1996). *Breastfeeding: a guide for midwives*. Books for Midwives Press, Cheshire.

Holland, B., Welch, A.A., Unwin, I.D., Buss, D.H., Paul, A.A., and Southgate, D.A.T. (1991). *McCance and Widdowson's The Composition of Foods*, (5th ed). The Royal of Society of Chemistry, Cambrige.

Kelnar, C.J.H. (ed.) (1995). *Childhood and adolescent diabetes*. Chapman and Hall Medical. London.

Lawrence, R.A. (1994). *Breastfeeding: a guide for the medical profession*, (4th ed). Mosby, St Louis.

National Diet and Nutrition Survey (1995). National Diet and Nutrition Survey: Children aged 1½ to 4½ years and nutrition survey. HMSO, London.

Royal College and Midwives (1991). *Successful breastfeeding—a practical guide for midwives*. Holywell Press, Oxford.

Scriver, C.R., Beaudet, A.L., Sly, W.S., and Volle, D. (ed.) (1989). *The metabolic basis of inherited disease*, (6th ed). McGraw Hill, New York.

Shaw, V. and Lawson, M. (1994). *Clinical paeditric dietetics*. Blackwell Scientific Publications, Oxford.

Thomas, B. (ed.) (1994). *Manual of dietetic practice*, (2nd ed). Blackwell Scientific Publications, Oxford.

Wharton, B.A. (1987). *Nutrition and feeding of preterm infants.* Blackwell Scientific Publications, Oxford.

Walker-Smith, J. (1987). *Practical paediatric gastroenterology.* Butterworths, London.

Queen, P.M. and Lang, C.E. (1993). *Handbook of pediatric nutrition.* Aspen Publishers, Maryland.

Self-help groups

Listed below are some of the self-help groups relating to nutritional issues discussed in this book.

Association of breastfeeding mothers
26, Hearnshaw Close, London, SE26 4TH.

Association for Spinabifida and Hydrocephalus (ASBAH)
ASBAH House, 42 Park Road, Peterborough PE1 2UQ.

British Diabetic Association
10 Queen Anne Street, London, W1M 0BD.

Children's Liver Disease Foundation (CHILD)
138 Digbeth, High Street, Birmingham, B5 6DR.

Coeliac Society
P.O. Box 220, High Wycombe, Bucks. HP11 2HY.

Cystic Fibrosis Research Trust
Alexandra House, 5 Blyth Road, Bromley, Kent BR1 3RS.

Down's Syndrome Association
155 Mitcham Road, Tooting, London SW17 9PG.

Eating Disorders Association
Sackville Place, 44 Magdalen Street, Norwich, Norfolk.

Family Heart Association
Wesley House, 7 High Street, Kidlington, Oxford OX5 2DH.

Hyperactive Children's Support Group
59, Meadowside, Angmering, West Sussex BN14 4BW.

La Leche League of Great Britian
PO Box BM 3424, London WC1 6XX.

MENCAP
123 Golden Lane, London EC1Y 0RT.

Migraine Trust
45 Great Ormond Street, London WC1N 3HD.

National Association of Colitis and Crohn's Disease
98A London Road, St Albans, Herts AL1 1NX.
National Childbirth Trust
Alexandra House, Oldham Terrace, London W3 6NH.
National Eczema Society
4 Tavistock Place, London WC1H GRA.
National Federation of Kidney Patients,
Acom Lodge, Woodsetts, Worksop, Notts S81 8AT.
National Federation of Kidney Patients' Association (NFKPA)
Swan House, The Street, Wickham Skeith, Eye, Suffolk.
National Information for Parents of Prematures, Education, Resources and Support (NIPPERS)
St Mary's Hospital, Praed Street, Paddington, London W2 1NY.
National Society for Phenylketonuria and Allied Disorders
7 Southfield close, Willen, Milton Keynes MK15 9LL.
Research Trust for Metabolic Diseases in Children Research (RTMDC)
Golden Gates Lodge, Weston Road, Crewe CW1 1XN.
SCOPE
12 Park Crescent, London W1N 4EQ.
Vegan Society
7 Battle Road, St Leonards-on-Sea, East Sussex TN37 7AA.
Vegetarian Society
Parkdale, Dunham Road, Altrincham, Cheshire WA14 4QG.

Organizations offering nutrition information

The organizations listed below are useful sources for nutrition information. The British Dietetic Association can provide information regarding dietetic contacts at a local level. Nutrition information can also be obtained from local dietetic departments in the hospital and community.
British Dietetic Association
7th Floor, Elizabeth House, 22 Suffolk Street, Queensway, Birmingham B1 1LS.

British Nutrition Foundation
   High Holborn House, 52/54 High Holborn, London WC1V 6RQ.
Health Education Authority
   Hamilton House, Mabledon Place, London WC1H 9TX.
National Dairy Council
   5–7 John Princes Street, London W1M 0AP.
Nutrition Society
   10 Cambridge Court, 210 Shepherds Bush Road, London W6 7NS.
Scottish Health Education Group
   Woodburn House, Canaan Lane, Edinburgh EH1 3DE.

Index

air swallowing 137
additives 180, 184–5
adolescence 70, 79–82, 103–4
afro- Caribbean, diets of 123–4
alcohol, in pregnancy 31–2
amino acids, in breast milk 25
    in inborn errors of metabolism 206,
        207, 212, 215
amylase in breast milk 26–7
anorexia nervosa 81
anthropometrics 1, 9
anthropometric ratios 11–14
appetite, control of 141, 191
atherosclerosis 88–9
    Barker hypothesis 87, 100–2
    blood lipids 90–1, 93
    causes 88–9
    COMA report 84, 95, 98
    dietary modification in 95–102
    fatty streaks 88
    muesli belt syndrome 61, 87, 121
    obesity 99, 187, 194
    plaque 88
    risk factors 89–90
    smoking 87, 88, 91
    and undernutrition 87, 101–2
azo dyes 180, 185

Barker hypothesis
    see atherosclerosis
beans
    toxins in 116
behavior problems
    in school children 77–9
    sucrose and 77–8
    colourings and preservatives and
        180, 185
    see also hyperactivity
bizarre diets 57
body mass index 11, 12, 13
bottle feeding 37–44
    difficult feeders 142–4

extra drinks and 43–4
errors in technique 142
    overconcentration 42
    overfeeding 141
    number of feeds 38, 42
    safety of 37
    sterilization 43
    underfeeding 141
    see also formulas; weaning
bottle feeding caries 67–8
bottle propping 142
breast feeding 15–37
    attachment 19–20
    benefits of 16
    complementary feeds 24–5
    contra-indications 16, 18
    duration 23–4, 36–7
    engorgement 129, 130
    HIV and 18
    hormonal control 20–1
    preterm infants 19, 28, 128–9
    positioning 21, 22, 23
    prevalence 15, 19
    retracted nipple 129
    'running out of milk' 130–1
    supplementary feeds 24–5
    weight loss 20, 24
    see also lactation; vitamin
        supplementation; weaning
breast milk
    drugs in 28–30
    environmental pollution 30–1
    Enzymes in 26–7, 28
    fatty acid content 27, 35
    nutritional composition 25–8
Bulimia nervosa 81

calcium
    foods high in 35
    in pregnancy 34
    in lactose intolerance 180
    in vegan diets 112, 113

cancer
  in childhood 243
  dietary factors in prevention 106–7
  nutrition support in 243
cardiovascular disease
  see atherosclerosis; hyperlipidemia
centile charts, *see* growth charts
child abuse
  cult diets 117, 120
  Munchhausen by proxy 169
  non-accidental injury 145–6
choking 140–1
cholesterol
  HDL 89, 90–1, 93
  LDL 89, 90–1, 93
coeliac disease 176–8
colic 136–7
colostrum 20
  composition of 25
  immunoglobulins in 25–6
COMA report 84, 95, 98
constipation
  in infancy 138–40
  in older children 63–5
cows' milk 41
  allergy 164, 165, 166–8
  intolerance 164, 165, 166–8
  introduction of 44
  semi-skimmed 53, 97
  skimmed 53, 97
Crohn's disease 236–7
cult diets 117
  macrobiotics 120
  fruitarians 120
cystic fibrosis 210–11
  dietary treatment 211
  prevalence 210

demand feeding 23, 38
dental caries 66–8, 74
diabetes mellitus 219–22
  carbohydrate exchanges 221
diarrhoea 154–61
  acute 154–9
  chronic intractable 160
  de retour 160
  toddler 60–3
dissatisfied baby 146–51
drugs in breast milk 28–30

eating habits
  of young children 50–68
  of school children 69–79
  of adolescents 79–82
eczema 163, 174–5
  dietary treatment 175–6
elimination diets, *see* exclusion diets
energy requirements
  in infancy 17
  in pregnancy 32, 33
  in lactation 33
  in young children 51
  in school children 70
  in adolescents 70
engorgement 129, 130
enteral tube feeding 225, 226, 227,
  229–33
epilepsy 222–3
ethnic diets 121–5
ewes' milk 38, 114, 168
exclusion diets 172–4

failure to thrive 61, 87, 121, 169, 228
  in breast fed babies 126–7
fats and oils, dietary 92, 95–7, 98–9
fatty acids
  in breast milk 27, 35
  in cardio-vascular disease 88–91,
   93
  deficiency 121
  in foods 92, 95–7, 98–9
  in infant formula 37
  ratio in diet 95, 98
feeding problem 126–52
feed thickeners 132–4
fibre 99
  high fibre diet 64–5
  foods high in 66, 99
folic acid 31
  and neural tube defects 31
  foods high in 32
  supplementation 31
follow-up milks 41, 44
food allergy 162–86
  acute reactions 164–5
  cows' milk protein 164, 165, 166–8
  diagnosis 168–71
  dietary treatment 171–4
  IgE in 163

peanut 165
prevention 164
wheat 165, 176–8
see also eczema
food challenges 169–71
food fads 54–7
food intolerance 135, 162–86
cows' milk 164, 165, 166–8
and hyperactivity 183–5
gluten 176–8
lactose 124, 159, 179–80
misdiagnosis 168, 183
undefined 182–5
migraine and 180–2
see also food allergy
food refusal 54–7
force feeding 145–6
foremilk 26
formulas, infant
animal fats in 113
composition of 39, 40, 41
dilution 42
infant
over concentration 42
preparation 42
pre-term 46, 48
special 167, 213
soya 113–15, 167, 179, 218
tube feeding 231, 232
whey v. casein based 37–8
formula switching 135, 137, 151
fruitarian 120

galactosaemia 216
dietary treatment 217–18
epimerase deficiency 218
galactokinase deficiency 218
prevalence 217
gastrostomy feeding 228, 229–33
gluten enteropathy, *see* coeliac
disease
glycogen storage disease 218–19
Goats' milk 38, 114, 168
Growth
in breast fed babies 20, 24, 126–7
monitoring 1–14
problems 9, 10–11, 126–7
in renal disease 238
reverting to the mean 10

in vegans 112, 117
Growth charts 3–8

haemagglutinins, in beans 116
health of the nation 85–7, 187
8 guidelines for a healthy diet 85
balance of good health 86
heart disease, *see* atherosclerosis
hiatus hernia 131
HIV 18, 241–2
Hydration 155–7
hyperalimentation, *see* parenteral
feeding
Hyperactivity 77–8
and food additives 184–5
and food intolerance 183–5
hypercholesterolaemia 93
dietary treatment 208–9
treatment 209
hyperlipidaemia 93, 208–10
hypernatraemia 42
hypertension
in afro-Caribbeans 94
salt and 94–5
hypoglycaemia 128–9, 220

Immunoglobulins 25–6, 163
inborn errors of metabolism
prevalence 206, 207
treatment 206
PKU 212–15
organic acidaemias 215–16
see also cystic fibrosis,
galactosaemia, glycogen storage
disease
Infant feeding 15–49, 126–52
Inflammatory bowel disease 236–7
iron
dietary sources 34, 60
in cows' milk 41, 44
in follow-up milks 41, 44
in pregnancy 34
iron deficiency 102–4
in asians 104, 123
in infants 103
in young children 57–8, 59, 72–3,
103
in adolescents 80, 103–4
in vegetarians 111, 113

Jainism 122
jaundice 128

Ketogenic diet in epilepsy 222–3

Lactation
    delay in establishment 127–8
    establishment 19–21
    fluid intake, and 35
    see also breast feeding
lactoferrin 26
lactose
    in breast milk 28
    intolerance 124, 159, 179–80
lipase, in breast milk 26–7
lipids, *see* cardiovascular disease
liver disease 234–6
lysosyme 26

macrobiotic diets 120
maternal diet 31–6
Methylmalonic acidaemia 215
migraine 180–1
    dietary management 181–2
    vasoactive amines 181
Munchausen by proxy 169

nephrotic syndrome 240–1
nitrates, in breast milk 31
nutrient needs
    in pregnancy 31–4
    in lactation 34–6
    in infants 17
    in young children 51, 70
    in adolescents 70
nutritional support, home 226–9

obesity 187–203
    behavior modification 191, 200–1
    cardiovascular risk factors 99, 187,
        194
    causes 189–93
    consequences 187, 193–5
    dietary treatment 195–200
    and exercise 188, 189–90, 199

family therapy 200–1
    in infancy 199–200
    prevalence 187, 188
    prevention 195, 201–3
    treatment 194, 195–200
oesophagitis 131, 162
olive oil 90, 92, 96
oral rehydration fluids 155–7
organic acidaemias 215–16
    dietary treatment 216
osteoporosis 105
Overconcentration of formulas 42
overfeeding, infants 135, 141

parenteral feeding 160, 225–6, 227,
    233–4
pesticides, in breast milk 30
Phenylketonuria 212
    dietary treatment 213–15
Pickwickian syndrome 194
possiting 131–4
Prader-Willi syndrome 193
Pre-term infants
    breast feeding 19, 28, 128–9
    formula feeding 37, 46, 48
    care in the community 46, 48
prolactin 20, 21
puberty 81

radiation
    in breast milk 30
    in formulas 30
Rastafarian diets 124
reference nutrient intakes (RNI)
    in infants 17
    in pregnancy and lactation 33
    in young children 51
    in school children 70
    in adolescents 70
renal disease 238–41
rickets 104–5, 122–3
rumination 135

school child, balanced diet and 69–72
school meals 75–7
smoking
    and atherosclerosis 87, 88, 91
    and vitamin C intake 34

snack foods 53, 54, 100
soya
    and cows' milk intolerance 167
    formulas 113–15, 167, 179, 218
    milks 38, 113
    oil 92, 93
special formulas 167, 213
special diets 109–25, 204–23
sterilizing agents 43
sucrose, and behaviour 77–8
sunflower oil 92, 96

tartrazine 180, 185
toddler diarrhoea 60–3
toddler diet 52–4
trans fatty acids 91
tropical oils 91, 92
trypsin inhibitors in beans 116
tube feeding
    enteral 225, 226, 227, 229–33
    parenteral 160, 225–6, 227, 233–4

ulcerative colitis 236–7
underfeeding, infants 141
undernutrition
    and atherosclerosis 87, 101–2
    and iron deficiency anaemia 102–4

Vasoactive amines in food 181
vegans 112, 113, 114

sources of "at risk nutrients" 114
vegetarian diets 110–17
    milk substitutes 113–15
    meal plan 118–19
    nutrient deficiencies 111, 112
    weaning 115–17
vitamins
    intake in school children 78–9
    prenatal storage 33–4
    toxicity 78
    welfare drops 36
vitamin supplementation
    in asians 123
    breast fed babies 36
    maternal 31, 34
    preschool child 57, 58–9
    in vegetarians 112, 116–17
vomiting 134–5
    habitual 135
    reflux 131–4

weaning 44–9, 146–50
    adding solids to bottle 45, 147
    breast fed babies 37, 45
    early introduction of solids 147
    menus 47
    vegetarians 115–17
weight reducing diets 195–200
wind 137–8

Z scores 14